Reiki Manual

Level One

Rajesh Nanoo

For orders and enquires, contact
www.rajeshnanoo.com
mrknowable@gmail.com

I, the Supreme Spirit,
Abiding in the body of living beings
As the Fire (Vaiswanara) in their stomach
I am associated
With their Praana and Apaana (Breathe),
Digest the four type of foods
(solids, fluids, semi-fluid and liquid)
Which they eat

Bhagavat Gita

Dr. Rajesh Nanoo MD(AM) had a spiritual inclination from my early days towards occult sciences and music. At first he nurtured his skills in Multimedia and started creating logos, posters and storyboard for various clients. Shortly his attention shifted to the potentials of Reiki and embraced this astonishing healing power. With enthusiasm, he pursued this magnificent profession along with Yoga Therapy and learned other holistic techniques which enabled him to hasten the healing process.

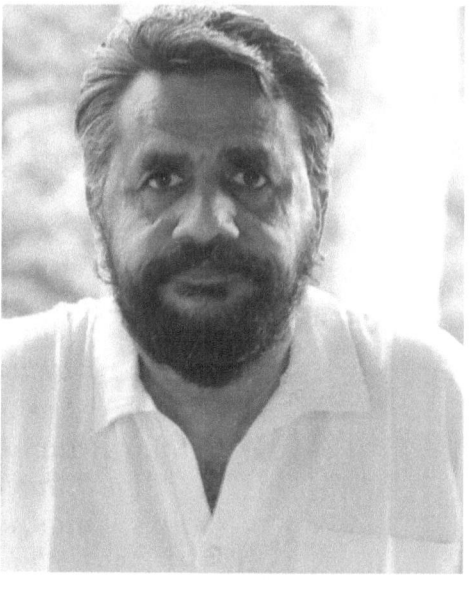

The research done on various philosophies enabled him to come up with training modules on enhancing life skills. He was involved in training people on the secret of working smartly, giving energy healing and teaching relaxation techniques to withstand the stress of the modern society.

Holistic training/healing methodology is a self-help tool to pull us out from difficulties; it has an integral part to play in character making. Rajesh Nanoo have comprehended this truth and crave to extend this awareness for the needy ones for cure and also to renovate their character, thereby let the world recognize the new era of healing/training that has begun by transcending a man completely.

CONTENTS

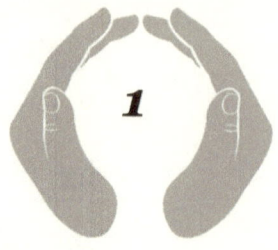

1   *Classification*

Alternative therapies and general medicines

1. Treatments by medication: (Allopathic or Modern Medicine, Ayurveda, Homeopathy, etc.)

2. Treatments without medication. (Reiki, Yoga, Acupressure, Reflexology, etc.)

All treatment modalities excluding Modern Medicine are called Alternative therapies. They are also mentioned as Complementary medicines, unorthodox medicines, Holistic medicines, Ethno medicines, and Natural medicines. In 1973, the medical faculty of the 'University of Rome' conveyed the first world congress of Alternative Medicines, and the provisional program contained more than 135 different therapies.

The World Health Organization (WHO) have also identified and enlisted more than 100 types of practices that they have defined as alternative medicines. Reiki has been recognized as an alternate therapy by the National Centre for Complementary and Alternative Medicine (NCCAM) at the US National Institute of Health (NIH).

NCCAM defines Reiki as – "Reiki" ("RAY-kee"). Reiki is a Japanese word representing Universal Life Energy. Reiki is based on the belief that when spiritual energy is channeled through a Reiki practitioner, the patient's spirit is healed, which in turn heals the physical body. Reiki appears to be generally safe, and no serious side effects have been reported". Reiki is rapidly acknowledged by most hospitals worldwide.

WHO also uses the term "Complementary Medicine" to describe "alternative Medicine". These terms are used interchangeably with "Traditional Medicine" in few well-known countries. Complementary/alternative medicine often refers to traditional medicine that is practiced in a country but is not part of the country's own traditions. As the terms "complementary" and "alternative" suggest, they are sometimes used to refer to health care that is considered supplementary to allopathic medicine.

However, this can be misleading. In some countries, the legal standing of complementary/alternative medicine is equivalent to that of Modern medicine. Many practitioners are certified in both complementary/alternative medicine and modern medicine, and the primary care provider for many patients is a complementary/alternative practitioner.

NCCAM describes complementary and alternative medicine as: *"a group of diverse medical and health care systems, practices, and products that are not presently considered to be part of conventional medicine."*

While some scientific evidence exists regarding some complementary and alternative medicine therapies, for most there are key questions that have yet to be answered. We may find answers through well-designed scientific studies, questions such as whether they are safe and whether they work for the diseases or medical conditions for which they are used.

These organizations also regard alternative medicines as a complementary to conventional medicine. The NCCAM states *"complementary medicine is used together with conventional medicine"*.

An example of a complementary therapy is by using aromatherapy to help lessen a patient's discomfort following surgery. Alternative medicine is used in place of conventional medicine. An example of an alternative therapy is by using a special diet to treat cancer, instead of undergoing surgery, radiation, or chemotherapy that has been recommended by a conventional doctor.

Authentic analysis

Even though Conventional medicine and the supportive organizations have nepotism and are trying to corner alternative medicine in their shed, but still the reality is far away from them. Alternative medicines have their own identity and at the same time can also be complementary. Increasingly, masses and doctors worldwide are shifting to alternative medicine as early as possible. Recent surveys affirm that 80% of people worldwide rely on alternative medicine. This swing is also accredited by the World Health Organization. It asserts,

"WHO supports traditional and alternative medicines when these have demonstrated benefits for the patient and minimal risks," said Dr Lee Jongwook, Director-General of WHO. "But as more people use these medicines, governments should have the tools to ensure all stakeholders have the best information about their benefits and their risks." It conveys further, "Empirical and scientific evidence exists to support the benefits of acupuncture, manual therapies and several medicinal plants for chronic or mild conditions". Alternative medicine not only deals with medicinal type treatments there are other healing modalities which never uses medicines for healing. They either use hands for healing (Reiki, Therapeutic Touch etc) or the body movements (yoga, Tai chi) to heal the diseases and they can be referred as Therapeutic activity. The WHO has accredited their achievement as genuine one. It suggest".

Therapeutic activity refers to the successful prevention, diagnosis and treatment of physical and mental illnesses; improvement of symptoms of illnesses; as well as beneficial alteration or regulation of the physical and mental status of the body.

The NCCAM classifies complementary and alternative medicine therapies into five categories, or domains as:

1. Alternative Medical Systems, which are built upon com-

plete systems of theory and practice. Often these systems have evolved apart from, and earlier than the conventional medical approach. Examples of alternative medical systems that have developed in Western cultures include homeopathic medicine and Naturopathic medicine. Examples of systems that have developed in non-Western cultures include traditional Chinese medicine and Ayurveda.

2. Mind-Body Interventions use a variety of techniques designed to enhance the mind's capacity to affect bodily function and symptoms. Some techniques that were considered as complementary or alternative medicine in the past have become mainstream, for example, patient support groups and cognitive-behavioral therapy. Other mind-body techniques are still considered complementary or alternative medicine, including meditation, prayer, mental healing, and therapies that use creative outlets such as art, music, or dance.

3. Biologically Based Therapies use substances found in nature, such as herbs, foods, and vitamins. Some examples include dietary supplements, herbal products, and the use of other so-called "natural" but as yet scientifically unproven therapies.

4. Manipulative and Body-Based Methods are based on manipulation and/or movement of one or more parts of the body. Some examples include chiropractic or osteopathic manipulation, and massage.

5. Energy Therapies: Energy therapies involve the use of energy fields. They are of two types:

1. Bio-field therapies are intended to affect energy fields that purportedly surround and penetrate the human body. The existence of such fields has not yet been scientifically proven. Some forms of energy therapy manipulate Bio-fields by applying pressure and/or manipulating the body by placing the hands in, or through, these fields. Examples include qi gong,

Reiki, and Therapeutic Touch.

2. Bio-Electromagnetic based therapies involve the unconventional use of electromagnetic fields, such as pulsed fields, magnetic fields, or alternating current or direct current fields.

Dynamic Categorizations

There are many alternative and complementary therapies. Many, but not all are listed below. This list is approved by NC-CAM.

Acupressure is the application of pressure using beads, seeds or other hard substances to specific pressure points that are associated with desired health benefits, such as weight loss, headache and pain relief, and even the disruptive symptoms of post-addictive withdrawal. It is derived from ancient eastern medicine, which defined the general principles of acupuncture points found throughout the body.

Acupuncture is one form of treatment utilized in the ancient medical practice of Traditional Chinese Medicine, the fundamental cornerstone and basis for the practice of Oriental Medicine, which balances energy levels in the body. Acupuncture uses fine needles that act like antenna to directly manipulate the body's energy levels.

The Alexander Technique is a method that works to change movement habits in everyday activities. It is a simple and practical method for improving ease and freedom of movement, balance, support and coordination. The technique teaches the use of the appropriate amount of effort for a particular activity, giving practitioners more energy for all activities. It is not a series of treatments or exercises, but rather a re-education of the mind and body.

Aromatherapy is the technique of using essential oils to relax, balance and stimulate the body, mind and spirit.

Auriculotherapy is a procedure in which stimulation of the auricle of the external ear is utilized to alleviate health conditions in other parts of the body.

Ayurveda places an emphasis on prevention and encourages the maintenance of health through close heed to a balance between right thinking, diet, lifestyle and the use of herbs.

Bach flower treatments are based on 38 remedies directed at a particular characteristic or emotional state.

Biofeedback is a training technique in which people are taught to improve their health and performance by using signals from their own bodies.

Chakra is a Sanskrit word meaning wheel, or vortex, and it refers to each of the seven energy centers of which the consciousness or energy system, is composed. The functioning of the non-physical chakras reflects decisions made in response to conditions encountered in life.

Chi Gung or Qi Gong (pinyin spelling) translates to "Energy Cultivation". There are several different styles of Chi Gung practiced in the world today. Probably the most widely practiced form of Chi Gung is a number of exercises designed to promote health and longevity, increase concentration, vitality and stamina, slow the aging process and enhance sexual functioning.

Chripractic manipulation is treatment using the therapist's hands to apply body leverage and a physical thrust to one joint or a group of related joints to restore joint and related tissue function. Through the use of manipulation, the aim is to provide relief from symptoms, improve joint and muscle function, and speed recovery. Spinal manipulation is the most common form of manipulation.

Colloidal Mineral Supplements are created by suspending minerals in pure water with an electronic colloidal process that creates liquid mineral suspensions.

Color Therapy uses the seven color of the spectrum to balance and enhance the body's energy centers or Chakras and also to help stimulate the body's own healing process.

Cranio-Sacral Therapy involves a very gentle touch of a practitioner's hands, both for diagnosis and for treatment. This light contact may be taken up on the cranium, the sacrum or any other part of the body as appropriate. Through this light touch the practitioner reportedly picks up subtle patterns of motion within the body.

Crystal Healing involves placing crystals of an appropriate color and energy at corresponding chakra points. It is reported that this process will cleanse and energize the chakras.

Dance or Movement Therapy is the psychotherapeutic use of movement as a process which furthers the emotional, cognitive, social and physical integration of the individual.

Dar' Shem is an ancient healing art in which the initiated reportedly channel energy through their bodies to help others.

Electrotherapy is the application of electricity to the human body in the treatment of disease.

The Feldenkrais Method is an educational system that develops a functional awareness of the self in the environment.

It is an approach to working with people which expands their repertoire of movements, enhances awareness, improves function and enables people to express themselves more fully.

Feng Shui is part of an ancient Chinese philosophy of nature and is often identified as a form of geomancy, divination by geographic features, but it is mainly concerned with understanding the relationships between nature and ourselves.

Gestalt Therapy is based on two ideas, the proper focus of psychology is the experiential present moment and we are inextricably caught in a web of relationship with all things. Its theory provides a system of concepts describing the structure and organization of living in terms of aware relations.

Hemi-Sync is a process that reportedly allows people to alter their brainwaves with multi-layered patterns of sound frequencies. When these sounds are heard the brain responds by producing a third, binaural, sound that encourages the desired brainwave activity.

Holotropic Breathwork combines accelerated breathing with evocative music in a special set and setting. A person uses their own breath and the music in the room to enter a non-ordinary state of consciousness.

Homeopathy or the way of similar, is a treatment approach where a person with a particular set of symptoms, is given a minute dose of a substance which in large doses causes similar symptoms in a healthy person.

Huna is system of psychology and religious methods long used by the Kahuna of ancient Hawaii, used to heal the sick, solving personal problems, untangling financial and social difficulties, and changing the future.

Hydrotherapy, or Water Therapy or Pool Therapy, consists of a variety of aquatic-based treatments that are designed to condition and strengthen muscles, and increase the range of motion in affected parts of the body by partially overcoming the effects of gravity with the buoyancy effect of the water.

Hypnosis is a subconscious condition in which the mind is more or less inactive and is sensitive to suggestions made by a hypnotist.

Iridology is the study of the iris of the eye in order to diagnose disease.

Karuna means any action that is taken to diminish the suffering of others and could also be translated as "compassionate action."

Kirlian photography records an image on a photographic plate of an object subjected to a high-voltage electric field. The image looks like a colored halo or coronal discharge. This image is said to be a physical manifestation of the spiritual aura or "life force" which allegedly surrounds each living thing.

Magnet therapy is based on claims that magnetic fields have healing powers, can help broken bones heal faster, and relieve pain.

Massage Therapy is used for relief from injuries and certain chronic and acute conditions, to help people deal with the stresses of daily life, and to maintain good health.

Meditation is a technique developed to achieve deep relaxation, eliminate stress, promote health, increase creativity and intelligence, and attain inner happiness.

Metamorphosis is a simple approach to healing and transformation in which the spinal reflex points on the feet, hands, head or directly on the spine are used to let go of the underlying genetic and karmic stresses brought in at conception.

Mindfulness is a type of meditation practice, known as vipassana, or insight meditation.

Movement Therapy or Dance Therapy is the psychotherapeutic use of movement as a process that furthers the emotional, cognitive, social and physical integration of the individual.

Music therapy is the prescribed use of music to bring about positive changes in the psychological, physical, cognitive, or social functioning of individuals with health or educational problems.

Naturopathy is a system of therapy and treatment which relies exclusively on natural remedies, such as sunlight, air, water, supplemented with diet and therapies such as massage.

Neuromuscular Integrative Action is a dynamic workout program that motivates people to achieve fitness, health, well-being, potential, and improved self-esteem.

Neuro-Linguistic Programming is a methodology used to explore how people organize their thinking processes, their beliefs and their behavior so that others can replicate their skills and capabilities in particular areas.

Nutraceuticals (often referred to as phytochemicals or functional foods) are natural, chemical compounds that reportedly have health promoting, disease preventing or medicinal properties.

Oriental Medicine includes the various styles that developed as Traditional Chinese Medicine spread from China to many different countries such as Korea, Japan and then into Europe. It uses ancient diagnostic techniques that evaluate and diagnose a person's imbalance. Once the patient is diagnosed, a treatment protocol using acupuncture, herbal prescriptions as well as other various modalities can be used.

Past Life Regression is the reported journeying into a person's past lives while hypnotized.

The Pilates Method is an exercise system focused on improving flexibility and strength for the total body without building bulk.

Polarity Therapy is a health system involving energy-based bodywork, diet, exercise and self-awareness. It works with the reported Human Energy Field, electromagnetic patterns expressed in mental, emotional and physical experience.

Pool Therapy, or Water Therapy or Hydrotherapy, consists of a variety of aquatic-based treatments that are designed to condition and strengthen muscles, and increase the range of motion in affected parts of the body by partially overcoming the effects of gravity with the buoyancy effect of the water.

Psychotherapy is a method of treating disorders, especially nervous disorders, by mental means rather than by using physical intervention techniques.

Qigong is the skill of cultivating internal energy using meditation techniques and external energy through movement patterns.

Reflexology is based on the concept that congestion or tension in any part of the foot mirrors congestion or tension in a corresponding part of the body. The reflex areas on the feet and hands are linked to other areas and organs of the body within the same zone.

Regression therapy is based on the concept that people are eternal beings who carry forward experiences and knowledge from one lifetime to another.

Reiki ("RAY-kee") is a Japanese word representing Universal Life Energy. Reiki is based on the belief that when spiritual energy is channeled through a Reiki practitioner, the patient's spirit is healed, which in turn heals the physical body

Rolfing, or Structural Integration, is a system of soft tissue manipulation and movement education that organisms the body in a way to ease pain and chronic stress, and improve physical performance.

Self-Hypnosis is a method of relaxation and introspection similar to meditation intended to attain a level of relaxation and concentration to allow a person's mind to send healing messages to their body.

Shamanism is a primitive religion in which it is believed that good and evil spirits pervade the world and can be influenced only by shamans acting as mediums.

Shiatsu is a traditional hands-on Japanese massage healing therapy to induce deep relaxation that can help in cases of specific injuries and for more general symptoms of poor health.

Sound Therapy examines the effects of low frequency sound and vibration on human health and wellbeing.

Spiritual Healing involves the concept of channeling healing energy from its spiritual source to someone who needs it. The channel is often a person, known as a healer, and the healing energy is usually transferred to the patient through the healer's hands. Praying can also be used to take advantage of spiritual healing.

Stress Management is the skill of dealing with the many stresses, including the psychological stresses of everyday living.

Structural Integration, or Rolfing, is a system of soft tissue manipulation and movement education that organisms the body in a way to ease pain and chronic stress, and improve physical performance.

Tai Chi, or Tai Chi Chuan, is an ancient Chinese form of coordinated body movements focusing on the cultivation of internal energy to harmonize the mind, body and spirit, promoting both mental and physical well-being through softness and relaxation. It is also an effective system of self-defense.

Taoist Healing is based on the concepts of a total body-mind-spiritual interaction according to theories explaining the balance of the complementary and antagonistic units which comprise the universe.

Thai Massage is an ancient method of aligning the energies of the body and originates from the time of the Buddha.

Touch Therapy, or healing touch therapy, encompasses a group of non-invasive techniques that utilize the hands to reportedly clear, energize, and balance human and environmental energy fields body to induce deep relaxation and promote self-healing.

Trance Dancing involves moving, breathing and concentration to express the rhythms of music to move energy from the body to other dancers.

Transpersonal Psychotherapy is a therapy combining western psychotherapies and eastern wisdom traditions.

Vedic Vibrations are traditionally believed to be fundamental vibrations that structure the material universe and the human body and reportedly generate "silent whispers" in people's consciousness which can be used to enliven the body's inner intelligence and bring immediate relief of symptoms of poor health.

Vibrational Therapy, or Vibrational Medicine and Energy Medicine, is based on the concept that all matter vibrates to a precise frequency and that by using resonant vibration, the balance of matter can be restored.

Vipassana which means to see things as they really are, is one of India's most ancient techniques of meditation.

Water Therapy, or Pool Therapy or Hydrotherapy, consists of a variety of aquatic-based treatments that are designed to condition and strengthen muscles, and increase the range of motion in affected parts of the body by partially overcoming the effects of gravity with the buoyancy effect of the water.

Yoga is a holistic system of self transformation that approaches well-being through balancing the vital energies in the body which harmonize all aspects of the physical, mental, emotional and spiritual aspects of human life.

Zen Buddhism is based on the teachings of Siddhartha Gautama, or Buddha, which contend that everything is subject to change and that suffering and discontentment are the result of attachment to circumstances and things which, by their nature, are impermanent. By ridding oneself of these attachments, including attachment to the false notion of self, people can be free of suffering.

Antiquity of healing

(Note: This article is published in Internet. It is written by Gloria Alvino R.Ph., B.S. in Pharmacy, M.S. in Health & Human Sciences, is founder & president of Heart to Heart Associates, Inc. a charitable, educational, non-profit organization.)

The science and art of medicine that was initially one, and then split into two, are now approaching reunion. The healing science that became traditional medicine and alternate medicine is slowly becoming the healing sciences. The history of this topic is extensive -- extending back thousands of years.

The history of medicine similarly reflects a fascination with the observation of the Human Energy Field (HEF) and its study. Back in 500 B.C., the Pythagoreans believed that, there is a universal energy pervading all of nature. They taught that its light could affect cures in sick patients.

In the 1100's, Liebault said that, humans have an energy that can react on someone else's energy, either at a distance or close by. According to Liebault, a person can have either an unhealthy or a healthy effect on someone else -- just by being present. The HEF of one person may be harmonious, or it may be discordant with another. The HEF of one person may be nurturing, or it may be draining to the HEF of another.

In the 1800's, Mesmer, the father of modern hypnotism, suggested that a field similar to an electromagnetic field might exist around the human body. Mesmer suggested that the power of this electromagnetic field, which he believed behaved as a fluid, might also be able to exert influence on the field of another.

In the mid-1800, Count Von Reichenbach spent 30 years experimenting with the human energy field, which he called the Odic field. He found that this field showed many properties which were similar to the electromagnetic field described by James Clark Maxwell in the early 1880's.

However, Von Reichenbach also showed that with the Odic force, like poles attract. In other words, like attracts like. In his work, "Physico physiological Researches on the Dynamics of Magnetism, Electricity, Heat, Light, Crystallization, and Chemism, In Their Relation to Vital Force", printed in New York in 1851, Von Reichenbach showed that electropositive elements gave his subjects feelings of warmth, and that this produced unpleasant feelings. In the reverse, electronegative elements produced cool and agreeable feelings.

He also found that the Odic field could be conducted through a wire. It traveled slowly at 13 feet per second. This speed depended on the density of the wire rather than its conductivity. He showed that part of this Odic field could be focused like a light through a lens, while another part of this Odic field would flow around the lens, like a candle flame flows around something placed in its path. Air currents would also move this part of the Odic field. This suggests a composition similar to a gas. Von Reichenbach's experiments suggest the Odic or Auric field is energetic, like a light wave, and also particulate, like a fluid. Also, he showed the right side of the body as being a positive pole, and the left as negative. This agrees with the ancient Chinese principles of yin and yang.

Carol L Norred-Although the scientific evaluation of spiritual healing is incunabular, anecdotes of healing by laying-on-of-hands predate written history. Psychic or intuitive healing by laying-on-of hands has been reported ancient Egypt. In 1550 B.C., the Ebers papyrus mentioned laying-on-of-hands for the relief of pain. In the sixth century, the physician philosopher Pythagoras described healing with energy or light surrounding the body. Often cited in the Bible, spiritual healings were performed by Jesus and three of his apostles: Ananias (Acts 9:1-19, 22:6-13), Peter (Acts 9:33-35), and Paul (Acts 9:36-41,14:8-10,16:16-19,20:9-12,28:3-6). Hippocrates theorized that a healing energy of nature was used with laying-on-of-hands. In the seventeenth century, Paracelcus reported a luminous sphere of energy surrounding humans and believed Etheric energy influenced by the mind affected the physical body.

Descartes believed that the mind could be separated from the body, leading to materialistic ontology in science. Supporting Descartes, Newton developed mathematics that reduced matter in the universe into atoms with absolute and linear time. Due to Cartesian influences upon modern science, theories of the paranormal that contradict conventional beliefs have been ignored or ridiculed within western orthodox medicine.

Patterson proposes that a human body may be considered interconnected and interrelated with everything in the universe. The work of physicist Albert Einstein removed the concept of a fixed and unchanging universe presenting that space and time are relative to the observer. The Newtonian view of absolute reality was proven incorrect by Einstein's quantum theory that postulates the universe is directed by a series of probabilities rather than fixed entities. Particles previously thought of as solid objects could be established to simultaneously act as both waves and particles existing in different space-time from normal experience. Recently physicist Stephen Hawking integrated a vision of unfixed relationships between space and time.

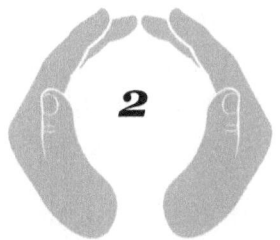

2   *Dr. MIKAO USUI*

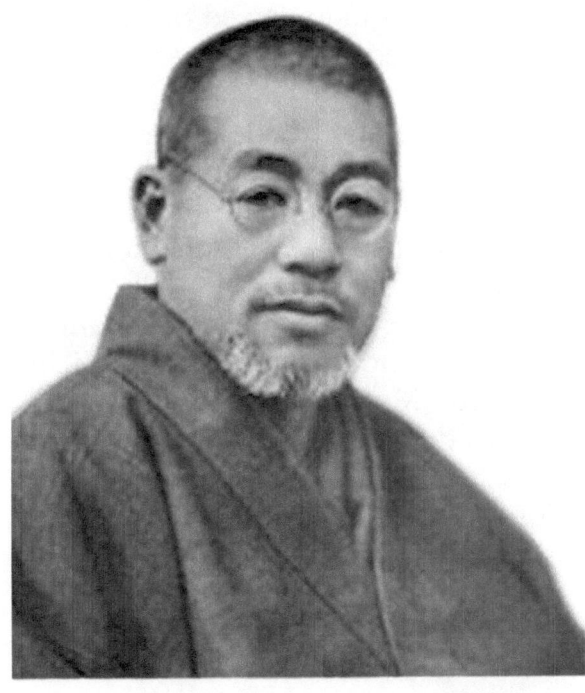

Dr Usui, or Usui Sensai, as he is called by his students in Japan, was born August 15, 1865. The Japanese word 'Sensei' means 'teacher, master, and doctor' and is a word generally used by students out of admiration for their teachers. It is not a title given or taken by one; rather it is given by a student as a sign of admiration for his teacher. The teacher would 'not at all' acquire or exploit the title himself.

The popular name of Usui is Mikao .He named his pen which was a very important Tool as Gyohan. He was born in Taniai-mura (now Miyama-cho) Yamagata-gun Gi- fu-ken, and had forefathers named Tsunetane Chiba who had played an active part as a military commander between the end of Heian Period and the beginning of Kamakura Period (1180-1230). His father was Uzaemon Tsunetane (a military commander) and his mother was from the Kawai family. Mikao Usui had three brothers, Sanya, Kuniji, and the third ones name is unknown. He also had an older sister called Tsuru. His family belonged to Tendai sect of Buddhism. He was married to Sadako, who hailed from the family background well known as Suzuki. Dr Usui had two children of his own, a son Fuji (1908-1946), and a daughter (name unknown 1913-1935).

As a child, he studied in a Tendai Buddhist monastery school at an early age may be at 4 years. Throughout his life, he was exceptionally spiritual and endowed the Buddhist tradition. At the age of 12 he practiced Martial Arts, in due course (approximately in mid-twenties) reached the highest levels of it. He did not stop there and studied several other ancient Japanese methods, and finally obtained high-level techniques in all his mastery in a short span of time. In his era, he was applauded by the most of the well-known martial artists.

He was friendly with several of Japan's famous teachers of Martial Arts, Jigoro Kano founder of Judo, Gichin Kuna- koshi founder of Karate, Morihei Ueshiba founder of Aikido and others. During this time he studied Qi Gong (called Ki-Ko in Japan, closely related to Reiki) to a high level and was able to do projection healing (When studying original Usui Reiki teachings, some of the techniques described are Qi-Gong techniques such as: Tapping Hand, Pushing Hand, and Stroking Hand, taught in Okuden or Second Degree Reiki).

It is believed that he meditated regularly at Kurama Yama. His memorial states that he was a talented, hardworking student, he liked to read and his knowledge of medicine, psychology, fortune telling and theology of religions around the world, including the Kyoten (Buddhist Bible) was vast.

Through his life experiences Usui-Sensei discovered the purpose of life was 'Anshin Ritsumei' or "The state of one's mind being totally in peace, knowing what to do with life, bothered by nothing". In India we call it "detachment". He intensely wanted to attain this state of mind, and hence he began his exploration. Distraught with his life and desperately seeking answers, he went to the Zen Master (guru as called in

India) and requested desperately how to realize it. He got the accurate reply "Die one time". These words motivated him to fast until he either die or became enlightened. He determined to fast on Mount Kurama Yama.

It is a sacrosanct mountain in Japan, Kurama means 'horse saddle' and Yama means 'mountain'. Mt. Kurama (570 Meters above sea level) is 12 kilometers due north of Kyoto Imperial Palace. The Kurama Temple, founded in 770 as 'the guardian of the northern quarter of the capital city' (Heian-kyo), is located halfway up the mountain. The original buildings have been frequently ruined by fire and subsequently reconstructed. The Main Hall was the last one to be restructured in 1971. The temple formerly belonged to the Tendai sect of Buddhism, but since 1949, it has been included in the newly founded Kurama-Kokyo sect as its headquarters.

At the time of Usui's fast, Kurama Yama was also the location of a spiritualist group called 'Rei Jyutsu Ka', which he may have also attended. He went to the mountain for the sole purpose to fast. It was not exceptional for Usui to fast as he made habitual trips to the mountain to seek answers. This is a common practice called 'Shyu gyo' a spiritual discipline, including the fast and meditation for 21 days, a strict spiritual training for advanced seekers. After 21 days, he became enlightened (or achieved Satori) and acquired healing ability. This healing system is known as Reiki.

The Reiki system was deep-seated in Tendai Buddhism and Shinto Buddhism. Tendai Buddhism (a form of mystical Buddhism) endowed with spiritual teachings, while Shintoism contributed techniques of controlling and functioning with the energies. As said earlier Usui be acquainted with both Kiko (energy cultivation) and a martial art and along with it had a strong Zen flavor (Yagyu Shinkage Ryu), and obtained Zen training.

During his study of Shinto and Mahayana (Mikkyo) Buddhism techniques he discovered Reiju (Empowerment method) and Hatsurei-ho (Cleansing process for body, mind and spirit). Another noted thing is the connection between

Usui's system and Shugendo (mountain asceticism). The core theme of that system was based on the Reiki principles. 'Real man grows with experience' therefore the knowledge obtained from these experiences will certainly ripe as a fruit while making his new system of healing.

He called it as 'Reiki Ryoho'. It was also often referred to as 'Usui Teate' or 'Usui hands-on healing'. Hand healing method is generally called as REIJIYUE-TUKA among Shinto Buddhist. Usui's teachings and techniques are called as 'Ronin' (leaderless) method. This was to ensure that none become a father who does not bear a Usui gene in their children's! Usui techniques will be bestowed to those who are genuinely needy. His system is called "USUI REIKI RYOHO".

The definition of Usui Shiki Ryoho in Japanese: 'Usui style healing method' or 'Usui system remedy' - the word Shiki means, 'system, method, form, rite, ceremony or style' and the word Ryoho means, 'healing method, therapy, remedy, and cure'. "Usui Reiki Ryoho" in Japanese is 'Usui spiritual energy healing method' which makes it more sensible. The word Natural does not appear (as in Usui System of Natural Healing).

It is believed that he was at the same time candid and controversial, and it caused apprehension among some of his friends. According to the reminiscence of one of his students - Sensei was very mild, gentle and humble by nature. He was physically big and strong. He did not accept fools willingly and could be quite harsh at times. He could get righteously angry and quite impatient, particularly with people who wanted results but were not prepared to work for that.

Can this behavior be termed as controversial? He always emphasized 'just for today' to all the queries. He was deadly against war, but liked the ancient 'warrior' sprit in individuals. He gave the masses spiritual lectures, practiced healing, and was spreading his knowledge and teachings about Reiki.

His method was a truly Spiritual one, which had a strong base on the Precepts. Students had to lead a proper life, healing themselves, emphasizing on health and happiness. Un- like today's Reiki teachings, meditation trainings were adapted for the revival and healing of one's own life and character. At that time, students firstly received the healing, from those who had genuine spirit to grasp this method and where initiated to the methodology of healing. This routine he followed at that time, was overall twisted by the modern masters while initiating Reiki now days. That ancient formula was the authentic approach to initiation and must be brought back.

The first record of Usui giving initiation (called Rei-ju) was in Harajuku, Tokyo in 1922. It was noted that, Initially Usui had no set hand positions; healing was done intuitively he also gave Reiki to those areas which had imbalances. (Painful areas). After- wards when he began teaching healing (Reiho) to others, he recognized the necessity to generate a set of instructions, which he called the "Usui Rei- ki Hikkei". Usui had a small manual which came into use about 1920 before he reached Tokyo.

After expounding Reiki, Usui pondered about spreading his techniques for the benefit of mankind and decisive to bestow it for the individuals. It is asserted in Usui Reiki Hikkei (one of his teaching manuals) Reiki should be spread to all, freely available up to the Shoden (first) level. Usui first practiced Reiki on his family and friends. It is said that Usui cured his wife with Reiki. The place was in fact Usui 's house; it had a banqueting hall, which was used for teaching and discussions. People were very poor in that area and they could not afford to consult a doctor. According to Japanese history articles, healing and other similar practices at that time would be given for very minimal cost, more likely for free. It is not yet known how his school was operated. We can only assume that it was very cheap or free to obtain healing at that time.

In April 1922, Usui founded Usui Reiki Ryoho Gakkai (Usui Reiki Healing Method Learning Society) and acted as its first president (this society still exists today). In 1923

September 1, shortly before noon, a great earthquake hit Tokyo and Yokohama, measuring 7.9 on the Richter scale. It destroyed the town, roughly killing 40,000 people and over 50,000 were seriously injured. Since Usui was living and working in the Tokyo area at that time, it is feasible that his school/home may also have been hit by the earthquake.

After that catastrophe, he was immersed in curing daily, going right through the inside and outside of the city. Ac- cording to his memorial status, during this disaster his way of availing help was to 'reach out his hands of love to suffering people'. His center was awfully tiny and did not have the competence to withhold the throng patients. This prompted him to construct a new abode in Nakano which is located outside the city. He switched to his new abode in February 1925.

An accurate or noted statistics are not available to date about the people who were rescued from death with his devoted healing from that fiasco. His devoted healing, in which he extended his hands of love to those tormented by this disaster, cannot be outlined and matched easily by the ones who have practiced healing. Due to his exemplary attitude displayed in the earthquake disaster, he was applauded with the coveted 'Kun San To' from the Emperor.

This lofty award (much like an honorary doctorate) is considered the best of its kind, which is solitarily awarded to those who have done incredible and applaud able endeavors. His exceptional healing skills along with fame escalated day by day throughout Japan, and this was ample enough to hasten the patients coming to his clinic for ailments. He also received numerous invitations throughout the country for Reiki training and healing after that.

Just prior to the earthquake, in order to meet the rising demand of healing from the public, Usui began to educate a simplified form of Reiki. This non-religious Reiki is termed as Western Reiki later on. While Usui was giving trainings to Reiki a few Naval Commanders - Ushida, Taketomi, Hayashi and others approached and requested to train them also.

There is a general assumption that they probably mastered the healing method and not the 'Spiritual Teachings' of Usui because of the short time. For this group he introduced a new phrase: 'Ryuku' was launched, its meaning can be defined as - someone who is an excellent practitioner but not recognizable with the full teachings.

An unclaimed figure of disciples of Usui is to be more than 2000; this massive list that includes the prime citizens inhabited in Tokyo to the common man. After his transition they mobbed at the training center and some of them pursued his work, while others absorbed in propagating Rei- ki healing. In 1926, a retired Rear Admiral Juzaburo Ushida (also pronounced Gyuda) became the chief of Usui Reiki Ryo- ho Gakkai. The other senior students of Usui including retired Rear Admiral Kanichi Taketomi and retired naval Captain Chujiro Hayashi were also assisting him. According to Hiroshi Doi (a member of Usui Reiki Ryoho Gakkai now) about 21(new research states it as 17 or 18) students were awarded Shinpiden (Master Degree) by Usui .

It was never unusual for Dr Usui to have a hec- tic schedule, as invitations for training of Reiki unrelenting- ly mounted up. He trekked right through Japan, which was a tough mission in those days. His constant travels may have made him tired. From Lama Yeshe's manuscripts, "Usui knew he would depart this life in a little while, thus he gathered all information, documents, observations, collection of holy Buddhist manuscripts, and his notes on Reiki in a box. He gave it to Watanabe, whom he considered his primary student and dearest friend". There is no proof or records at present of such mentioned handover, which had taken into action.

After a period of short time Usui toured Kure, Hiroshima, and Fukuyama with his close to heart sacred teachings. The final stage was set; the curtain of his Spiritual Healing life was drawing to an end. On March 9, 1926 while in Fukuyama at the age of 61, Usui had a fatal stroke and made the "transition"(Reiki's expression for passing on or dying) it is assumed that he practiced Reiki for long on the night before he breathed his last breath. After the cremation, his ashes were placed in a Temple at Tokyo. Shortly after his transition, students from Reiki society in Tokyo erected a memorial stone at Saihoji Temple in the Toyatama district in Tokyo in his fond memory.

Chujiro Hayashi was the celebrated person who accepted Usui's work loyally. This admired personality ignited the candle of Reiki for the future so it wouldn't be blown out after Usui's transition. He is called as the second father of Reiki because of this torch bearing. There is an argument that the word 'Reiki' was not created by Usui, and it was more exactly introduced by Hayashi or the other naval officers along with him. As said earlier, Usui's healing method has been referred to as 'Usui Teate' meaning 'Usui Hand Touch' or 'Usui Do'. In Usui's manual, the word "Reiki" in kanji language was not at all mentioned as a name of his system, but it can be noticed more on common scripts of the Hayashi manuals, and this support the doubt of that argument that Reiki was more Hayashi's term than that of Usui .

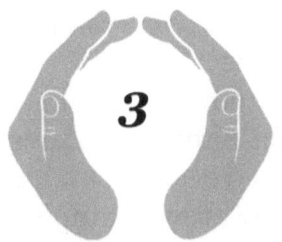

3   *CHUJIRO HAYASHI*

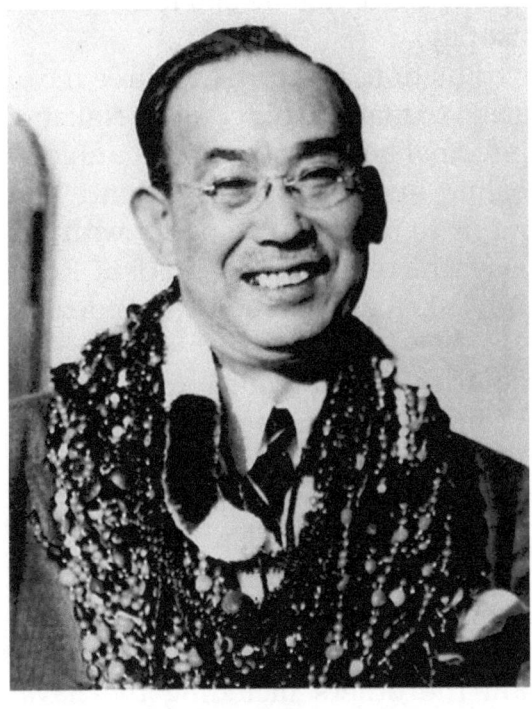

Dr Hayashi was born in 1878. He graduated from Navy School in Dec 1902. He had undergone medical train- ing, which included Eastern teachings (Chinese Medicine). He was appointed as Naval Doctor and later on as ex-naval 'Captain' in the Imperial Japanese Navy. He was one of the earliest non-Buddhist disciples of Usui . Usui trained him in late 1925 at the age of 47. It is believed he was trained along with the other naval officers Ushida and Taketomi. Hayashi's sojourn with his mentor lasted only for six months, as Usui subsequently made his transition.

When Hayashi started his training with Usui , very shortly, Usui recognized the character of Hayashi. Hayshi was a mortal made of solid principles and nevertheless was a Methodist Christian. He was unable to comprehend the mystifying nature of 'Usui Teate' because of Buddhist methodology. Subsequently, Usui altered the teachings so as to suit Hayashi. There is an idea that Hayashi did not acquire

Reiju (empowerment). So perhaps Usui imparted them (Hayashi and other naval officers) an innovative system of empowerment which was not practiced earlier.

Hayashi entitled this method of empowerment as 'Trans- formations'; the modern era again altered the given name as attunement or initiation. He mastered every technique, which was imparted to him by Usui and awarded Shinpiden maybe for his appreciative skills or as an acknowledgment of Hayashi learning, and not in the sense that he had mastered all Usui 's teachings and philosophy.

After the mentor's transition, in April, the three naval officers of Usui's school started to manage his clinic at Nakano, near Tokyo. According to informal hearsay, the hospice abided efficiently for 8 years; healing and teaching were part and parcel of this endeavor, and in 1931, due to disparity with the chairperson (Taketomi), Hayashi relinquished it (Usui Reiki Ryoho Gakkai). Ushida and Taketomi pursued the endeavor with the society.

Hayashi seized mentor's clinic, which was initially labeled as Usui Memorial Clinic and renamed it as 'Hayashi Reiki Kenkyuukai' or Hayashi Reiki Research Society. According to one of his prominent disciple's (Takatai) certificate, Hayashi entitled his system as 'Usui Reiki system of drugless healing'. According to another informal hearsay - when Hayashi made that significant change in the name, which may have an impact in altering the original teaching style also, owing to this apprehension the others including the naval officers relinquished Dr. Hayashi's school.

Mrs Hawayo Takata, was one of the major disciples of Hayashi sensei and the most prominent one who promulgated Reiki worldwide. She attained the Shoden level in 1935. She along with her 2 daughters stayed with the Hayashi's family in Japan for more than a year. In 1936 May; an excerpt from Takata's diary: "Mr Hayashi has granted to bestow upon me the secret of Shinpiden - Kokiyou-ho and Leiji-ho (Reiji) - the utmost secret in the energy science".

In 1937 - Before Takata left for Hawaii, she attended Hayashi's Okuden level class. There is a meek picture of a Hayashi Sensei and Mrs Takata's meeting with the title Reiki Ryoho ho Kai, 1937. At the bottom of the photo contains these words written in Japanese Kanji 'Reiki Ryoho Koushu Kai', the translation is 'Reiki Ryoho Training Meeting'. Hayashi Sensei also called the system as 'Usui Reiki Ryoho' as taught by Usui .

In 1938: February 21st, Hayashi officially conferred the title of Reiki Master Degree to Takata. Thus, she became a Reiki Teacher or Shinpiden. On the certificate of Takata, the name of the system is mentioned several times but all those names stated are different like: 'Usui system of Reiki healing', 'Usui Reiki system of drugless healing' and 'Dr. Usui's Reiki system of healing'. The first-degree certificate entitled as 'Usui Shiki Reiki Ryoho', second degree entitled as 'Usui Reiki Ryoho' and third degree entitled as 'Dr. Usui's Reiki Ryoho'. Hence, the system does not refer to Hayashi Shiki Ryoho (Ha-yashi style healing method) anywhere as his system of treatment and the other significant aspect to be noted is the word Reiki was used in all occurrences.

There is also a different story. Ms. Chiyoko Yamaguchi (a teacher of Reiki Ryoho learned from Dr. Hayashi) referred that their healing system was Hayashi-Shiki Reiki Ryoho (Ha-yashi style Reiki Healing Method). She currently teaches the way she says she learned, - Shoden and Okuden are taught during a 5 day workshop and Teacher level one month later. She does not refer to the Teacher level as Shinpiden because she does not think Hayashi Sensei called it by that name. The certificate Hayashi Sensei issued to her, has the name Hayashi Reiki Ryoho Kenkyu-kai (Research Centre) on it.

In the book 'The Reiki Healing' by Fuminori Aoki (master of Reido Reiki) Ms. Yamaguchi is quoted as saying, "I am not sure but it can be possible that Hayashi's teaching method was different between teaching in his clinic in Tokyo and going out of Tokyo to teach". She also said that she was not taught any formal hand positions.

This may be because Hayashi altered his methods by the time Yamaguchi took her training with him in 1938, or perhaps the methodology of Hayashi was to train each one according to their ability to withstand this great elusive energy, and as it seems, they do in the Gakkai. Hence most probably, Hayashi did not mention his system as Hayashi Shiki Ryoho (Hayashi Style Healing Method) rather than others who took training with Hayashi Sensei may have referred this name to that system.

Hayashi Sensei had numerous novel ideas, which were rapidly transcended to the structure of Reiki. He introduced the system of "degrees" and developed divergent supplementary hand positions suitable for clinical use. This massive contribution of codifying the hand positions for a full body treatment bestowed to the modern Reiki by this wizard cannot be under- estimated. He launched group healing into Reiki Treatment. Group healing method constitute of bundle practitioners join as a group to heal a single patient at the same time. If their mind and hands blend single heartedly then this method enhances the energy surge to a great extent.

Hayashi's clinic comprised eight beds and 16 healers. Two practitioners attended each patient. He modified some of the formats used by Usui . It is assumed that initially Hayashi used seven or eight hand positions, and covered the upper body only and these hand positions are embedded in the Eastern traditional healing techniques (such as Chinese Medicine).

According to this traditional healing methodology, the head and torso are the most vital elements of the body, and limbs are only "external" elements. The head and torso are vital because they are the foremost energy centers or meridian (acupuncture) points in our body, so while treating these areas, the energy will surge throughout the body including the arms and legs (via meridians). Hayashi Sensei believed it is only necessary to treat these vital points 'head and torso' and thereby, the energy will surge through the entire body and also to the subtler levels.

Usui also acquainted with this technique (head and torso) and healed in a similar way in most cases, but with exceptions. In those exceptional cases, further treatment was given mainly to the affected region. It is assumed that further treatment to the affected region was implemented in the later years of his life. It seems that Hayashi adoringly pursued this technique from his mentor and during the course of time came up with additional hand placements covering the entire body. This new technique endowed him with an enhanced surge of energy throughout the body quickly, rather than Usui's technique.

The first degree (Shoden) was awarded in a 5-day workshop either for a relatively high fee, or on an agreement that the student should associate with him as a healer for the fee. It is believed that student should work at least 8 hours per week for 3 months for Shoden and 8 hours per week for 9 months for Okuden (second degree). Hayashi Sensei gave his own manual called 'Ryoho Shishin' (Healing Method Guideline) to Shoden students. Hayashi's manual had 40 pages written in old style of Japanese kanji. In the advanced level of training he permitted the aspirants even to copy his personal remarks also.

The manual Hayashi gave to his students bares the identical name Usui used for the 'guideline section' of his Hikkei; this similarity is not limited just in name but also alike in the content and facade, they also enclose suggested positions for treating different maladies. Recent research reveals that, the basis why Hayash's manual became identical to Usui's, was because he asked Hayashi to provide a manual depicting hand positions for treating different ailments.

Hayashi may also probably have added several other chapters related to Reiki. He may have supplemented the knowledge that, Tatsumi San received information from Hayashi referencing Chinese Medicine, including a series of 7 hand positions that worked with the meridians. This statement most probably will not be true because this information does not agree with the content enclosed in Hayashi's manual, and also it seems that his major disciple Takatai did not receive this information!

The Second World War shattered the relationship between Japan and the United States. Hayashi Sensei in an intuition glimpsed the mammoth of terror that would swallow Japan in the outcome of war, and sooner or later as a reserve naval officer, he anticipated a call from authorities to play a part in the war. As a philanthropist his empathetic mind could not comprehend this barbaric act. His conscious mind gave the command to refrain from the war even by transition. Thus in 1940, Takatai received a telegraph from Hayashi demanding her to reach the clinic instantaneously.

On May 10th, addressing a short assembly of his Shinpiden students and family, Hayashi revealed that, as a cordial mortal it is weird in taking part in the war which was about to begin. He was geared up to transition and the clemency of this splendid healing tradition was bestowed to Takatai. He made his transition at the age of 62 on May 10-1940. He curtailed life by 'Seppuku' (Ritual splitting of the Hara). Hayashi had attuned 17 Reiki Masters according to Mrs Takata.

Mrs Hayashi sustained to teach Reiki in Japan after his transition and Mrs Takata (13th Shinpiden student) circulated the divine energy healing system throughout the world where as Mrs Yamaguchi pursued to teach Reiki Ryoho in Japan, and she never trained anybody publicly.

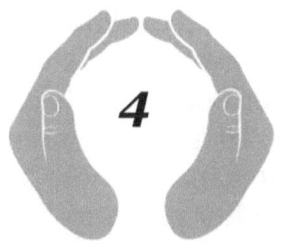

4   *HAWAYO TAKATA*

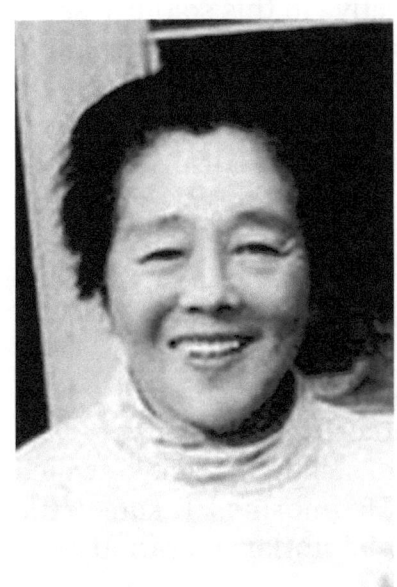

Hawayo Kawamuru (later known as Hawayo Takata), was born on December 24-1900, in the Hanamaulu, Kau- ai, Hawaii (U.S. territory of Hawaii). Mr and Mrs Otogoro Kawamuru, her parents, were sugar cane workers and immigrants. She grew up in a blended atmosphere of both cultures (Western as well as Japanese). She had a wretched childhood, which forced her to labor in diversely fields, as a sugar cane in a rich family. It is believed that she worked for this affluent family for about 25 years.

In the meantime she met her companion Saichi Takata and tied knots in 1917, March. She gave birth to two daughters (one named Alice Takata-Furumoto, who later had a daughter named Phyllis Lei Furumoto). The honey in her life was soon veiled by the clouds of terrors which start to blow one by one. Takata's husband Saichi Takata rescued to Japan for treating his chronic maladies but did not withhold it and soon passed away (October of 1930) at age 34 in Japan. This sobering incident was only a tip of iceberg and a few more was augmenting to blossom.

Takata was not willing to give up, brushed her grief aside and endeavored to labor extensive hours to endow with her family. This over burden affected the health and shortly various maladies began to creep into her body. She began experiencing abdominal pain and asthma. In 1935 her sister passed away, forcing her to take a voyage to Japan (where her parents were for a year-long visit) to inform her parents about this tragedy.

There also was another objective in this sojourn, seeking treatment for her asthma and abdominal pain. She, along with her sister-in-law, took a steamship and reached Japan. Hospital authorities diagnosed that, she had colon cancer, gallstones, inflamed appendicitis and other disorders. An operation was fixed as the remedy. A short interval of rest was allotted before operation for primarily recouping her strength. On the way to the Operation Theatre for a serious surgery, she heard an anonymous voice telling her that the operation was not essential.

In this uncertainty she requested her surgeon for an alternative method of curing her other than the surgery. As the doctor had a hint about Hayashi's clinic in Tokyo, which applies, innovate ideas for healing. He informed Takata of his knowing and belief which can be taken into consideration as an alternate to the appointed Surgery.

Her maiden debut with Hayashi's clinic was in 1935. She pursued treatment with two Reiki channels. In the progression of treatment, her curiosity in the Reiki system was amplified when the channels (healers) used to demonstrate those areas in the body where energy had a deficiency, these points were also similar to the problematic areas mentioned to her by the previous doctors. She was amazed by intense heat exuded from the healer's hands, and at a point of time she actually had a notion that some sort of equipment's which generates fervors is secretly enclosed beneath the outfit of healers and this instrument may be applied while healing. Thus healers in the Hayashi Sensei's clinic came under her scrutiny.

One day she snatched the sleeves of the healer but the endeavor to discover the instrument was futile. The astounded healer inquired about this scrutiny and when she expressed her reservations, which ended in a huge laugh. The Reiki healing methods stunned her. Their answers quenched her reservation. She was salvaged from the excruciating pain of her ailments by this fabulous energy in four months.

As stated earlier Takata was dumbfounded by the healing power of Reiki and became zealous to learn it. Hayashi was not solicitous to succumb to the appeal because of stern ethos. The major hurdle was Takata was a woman and also a resident outside Japan. It is believed that, during that time there was a suggestion that Reiki not ought to be taught outside Japan. It precisely means, a foreigner cannot acquire Reiki training. Again and again she pleaded with Hayashi and again and again he ridiculed her appeal. At last after a great deal compulsion from the surgeon (who recommended her to Hayashi) finally made her dream come true.

In the spring of 1936, Mrs Takata received Reiki First Degree. She associated with Hayashi for one year and then received Second Degree. Mrs Takata then returned to Hawaii in 1937. A few weeks later, Dr. Hayashi and his daughter arrived at Hawaii and stayed until February 1938 to establish Reiki healing system in her town. They also collectively gave several seminars.

In 1938, February 21, Takata was blessed with the coveted title of Reiki Shinpiden (Master). She was the thirteenth and last Reiki Master Hayashi Sensei initiated. When asked about Mrs Takata's fee for mastership training, Helen Haberly, (one of her students and author of 'Reiki, Hawayo Takata's Story') responded, "Mrs Takata had to put her house up for sale to pay for her Shinpiden training". We don't have any valid evidence to prove this statement as valid or invalid.

After Hayashi's transition, Takatai returned to Hawaii to get her belongings. Her plan was to reside in Japan and facilitate the endeavor at Hayashi's clinic in Tokyo. The Second World War constrained the liberty of immigrants to travel;

hence she as an immigrant was enforced to abode in Hawaii. Later at the end of the war she had the opportunity to revisit Japan. In her sojourn, she observed the unusual havoc of Japan, which had been totally dismantled by merciless bombarding. It is assumed that the only building that withheld the shattering of the war was the Reiki clinic.

In the meantime, Hayashi widow had altered the clinic into a refuge hub mainly for the downtrodden and also for youthful women. After pondering this issue, they came into the conclusion that Takatai would relocate to Hawaii and the widow would continue to manage the clinic.

Takatai first resided in Kauai, the big island (Hawaii), and later moved to Oahu. The aftermath of Second World War was somber, and in that agony, she as an archangel uplifted and pacified the world with her composed heart and lofty hands. Shortly a healing center was launched and later on was sold out when she shifted to Oahu again. Her span of healing and initiating islanders embarked for more than thirty years.

It is assumed that, she was reluctant to give master degree in those years and trained them only for first and second degree. Takatai mentioned her system in the same name as Usui and Hayashi called - Usui Reiki Ryoho. While issuing certificates to disciples she altered it slightly as 'Usui Shiki Ryoho' or ('The Usui System of Natural Healing').

After a while, she was invited to America to take a class on the First Degree. This was a turning point in the history of Reiki; it upsurge both, Takata as well as Reiki. This significant swing implanted the seed of Reiki to flourish globally. Takatai's became popular and there was an enormous rush to study Reiki internationally. She began to confer master degree initiation during this trip from Hawaii to America.

She realized the need to transmit the sacrosanct wisdom, so began training Reiki Masters between 1970 and 1980. She had a hectic schedule, which covered entire USA with her sacred teachings. When the honey is distributed bees rush from everywhere, similarly when she spread Reiki to those who felt sincere and worthwhile, students from different sides of globe started to throng in.

On a tape recording made during a class in 1979, Takatai told the history of Reiki and said that she learned 'Usui Reiki Ryoho' from Dr. Hayashi Sensei, which is the same name that Usui had mentioned. She added that there is neither deviation nor shrinking in the system, because Hayashi taught her exactly what he learned from Usui and the same substance is transmitted without any amendments. It is assumed that, (in 1976) she charged US$125 for First Degree (Shoden), US $400 or Second Degree (Okuden) and US $10,000 for Master Degree (Shinpiden).

She also employed another approach in which fees was charged according to the salary basis. One-week salary was charged for first degree and one month salary for second degree and one year salary for master degree. It should be noted that all of her master students did not pay the $10,000 fee. From an Internet site it's heard that- a master who paid $1,000 plus, he also sponsored a number of Mrs Takata's classes in exchange for the balance of the fee. The site says that another student Virginia Samdahl, Ethel Lombardi and Barbara Weber (Ray) sponsored numerous classes for Mrs Takata; perhaps in exchange for some or their entire Master ship fee.

Takatai initiated 22 or 23 Reiki Masters. The number always varied, but apparently she initiated as many as 22 individuals as Reiki Masters during her last decade of life. It is not known when Takatai made her sister Kay (a Reiki Master) may be a little bit earlier, (before 1970) all other Reiki masters were initiated after 1970. The reason she did not initiate masters before 1970 is an enigma and has not been revealed yet.

Dr. Barbara Ray, a student of Takata says : In the few years prior to her death, she did allow a few people to teach "The First Degree". However, true to her tradition of maintaining silence and protection, she did not disclose the details of the entire Usui system to anyone else. Most often when she taught someone The First Degree, she did not mention that there was a Second Degree. In addition, from the very beginning of her training and teachings, she requested them that while she was living, not to discuss or print anything regarding the entire system, and also not to initiate any Masters.

Now her noble mission almost came to anti-climax because Reiki became propitious in international stature as an indispensable healing technique for mankind. In this gusto, Takatai made her transition on December11-1940 at the age of 80.

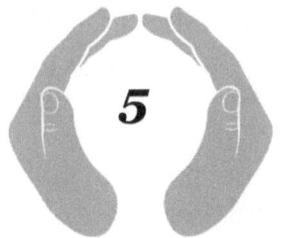

5   *Narration Of Events*

This information is obtained from William Lee Rand's website. This is a transcript of a tape recording of Mrs. Hawayo Takata telling some students about the history of Reiki. The recording was made in 1979 when Mrs. Takata was 78 years old. This was a year and a half before her transition. The tape, from which this transcript was taken, Mrs. Takata Talks about Reiki, can be ordered. This transcript is presented as part of The True History of Reiki research project, which supports efforts to investigate, collect, and share information about the historical roots of Reiki and its relation to others systems of healing. Through historical research, some of the details in the story below have been shown to be inaccurate. For a discussion of some of these historical details, see an Autumn 1996 article "The Original Reiki Ideals" in *Reiki,* "Was Dr. Usui a Christian?" in the first chapter of *Reiki, The Healing Touch* by William Rand. The most up to date information is now available in The Spirit of Reiki written by William Lee Rand, Walter Lubeck and Arjava Petter.

Takatai's narration

This is the story of Dr. Mikao Usui who is the originator of the Usui Reiki Ryoho. That is in Japanese, which means the Usui Reiki system of natural healing. At this time in the beginning of the story Dr. Usui was the principal of the Doshisha University in Kyoto. Also, minister on Sundays, and at the University they had a chapel. So he was a full-fledged Christian minister and my teacher was Dr. Hayashi, who was his pupil, and also he carried on the work after Dr. Usui 's passing.

So in other words Dr. Chujiro Hayashi was his 1 disciple, and this is through Dr. Hayashi that I have learned about Dr. Usui . I have never met him and he said that Dr. Usui was a genius, very, very brilliant, intelligent - a great philosopher and a great scholar.

One day, on Sunday, he was at the podium giving Sunday service- a lecture and that day he found there were about a half dozen students on the front pew. Usually the students of the University sit in the back. Then he said, "Good morning, everybody, I am going to deliver our regular Sunday sermon." Then one of the boys raised his hand and he recognized him, and he said "Yes, what is it?" and this young man said:

"We who are sitting here are some of the graduate students which are going to in two months- will be leaving this school; we'll be graduating [from] this University. But we would like to know for our future, whether you have absolute faith in the Bible." And Dr. Usui said "Certainly! I do! And that is why I'm a minister and I accept the Bible as it reads." So Dr. Usui was surprised to be asked. And then the boy said, "I represent this group, this graduating class and we would like to know more about your faith. Is it because you absolutely have faith in the Bible that you accept the Bible as written?" And he said "Yes, of all I have faith. And also I have studied the Bible and therefore, I believe."

Then the boy said, "Dr. Usui , we are young people in our twenties and we have a very big future. And we would like to clear this once and for all –and if you have so much faith in Christianity, should I believe and [do] you believe that Christ was able to heal by laying on hands?" And Dr. Usui said, "Yes, I believe." Then the boy said, "We would like to believe as you do, we would like to have that kind of a faith but we ask you, you are our great master and great teacher. We honor you and we respect you. Please, give us one demonstration." So Dr. Usui said, "What kind of a demonstration?" He said, "We'd like to see you heal the blind or heal the lame or walk on the water." And Dr. Usui said, "Although I am a good Christian and I have faith and I accept the Bible as it is, and I know Christ did it, but

I cannot demonstrate because I did not learn how to do it." So the boys said, "Thank you very much.

Now we shall choose our way and what we believe in. We can only say that your belief in the Bible is a blind faith, and we do not want to have blind faith, and then to live all our lives, we want at least to see one demonstration so that we will be able to follow you, and accept and to have faith like you." So Dr. Usui said, "Well, this I cannot demonstrate at this time. Let us not argue about it but some day I would like to prove it to you. And when I find the way I shall come back and I shall show you and I can demonstrate, I hope. And with this, I resign as of now. Immediately I will step down and I will put in my resignation as minister of Doshisha and also [as] principal of this University. Tomorrow being Monday, I shall start on a visa. And I shall go to a Christian country to study the Bible, and to study Christianity in a Christian country. And I might find the answer. And when I do, I shall come back. And I shall let you know that I can do what you have requested." And he said "good-bye". And he left the church as of that time.

And next day Dr. Usui started to apply for a visa, and he chose America. And when this was all done, he took the boat, and he came and traveled by train, and he entered the University of Chicago. He studied philosophy, but number one, he wanted to study Christianity and also the Bible. And when he went to the studies in America, he found that the Bible and the Christian school that he went to were identical, the teachings were the same. And he could not find in the Christian Bible even in America where Christ had left a formula for the healing. So being in this University where they had philosophies of the world, he went into other philosophies. He studied Hinduism, Zoroastrianism and of course, religion.

When he came into Buddhism he found a passage where it said that Buddha healed by laying on the hands. He healed the blind, tuberculosis, and also leprosy. When he found this out he said "I should further my studies in Buddhism and to find out whether Buddha has left any kind of a formula for the healing art." So Dr. Usui spent seven years in the United States and then he said, "It is time for me to go back to a Buddhist country and to study Buddhism and find the formula."

When he arrived in Japan he did not waste any time. He landed in Kyoto, where he lived before, and he went to all the great monasteries, and even today Kyoto is a Mecca of temples and it is the seat. At that time Nara was the seat of Buddhism but Kyoto had the most people and the biggest monasteries in Japan. And so he decided to visit to every single one. So, he started with the most biggest temple, the Shin and when he arrived there he met a monk, and he said "does the Buddhist bible or the Sutras, do the Sutras say that Buddha healed? Is it written down in the Sutras that Buddha had healed leprosy, tuberculosis, and the blind, by laying on of hands?" And the monk answered, he said "Yes, it is written in the Sutras." He said, "Have you mastered the art, can you do it?" And the monk said, "Well, in Buddhism, physical is very important, but we consider the church, or ministry, is to minister the people so they have better minds. We want to straighten their minds first so they'll become more spiritual and then show more gratitude and learn all, the better things of life. And this is a temple or a church, and we monks do not have time for the physical in reaching the spiritual growth, spiritual healing is first."

Dr. Usui bowed and said, "Thank you." And he walked away and he went to the, [to] Kyoto. Then he went also to the different temples and everyone had the same answer. They said "Yes, it is registered in the Sutras, and therefore we accept and we believe that Buddha was a healer. But, we are trying to heal the mind first, and therefore we do not know anything about healing the body."

After days and days and months of search Dr. Usui was very depressed. But he did not give up. He said, "I have one more place to go." And finally he learned it in a Zen temple. And when he approached the temple, he rang the bell, and a little page boy came out. And he said "I would like to speak to the highest monk of this Grand Temple." He said, "Please come in. And who are you?" And he said, "I am Mikao Usui . And I would like to study Buddhism, and therefore I would like to meet the monk." So the message was delivered, and when the monk came out, he was about a seventy-two-year-old monk, very lovely face like a child, innocent-looking, beautiful face, kindly voice, and very gentle and he said, "Come in. And so you are interested in Buddhism."

He said "Yes, but first, I would like to ask you a question. Does the Zen believe in healing?" He said, "Yes, we do. It is written in the Sutras that the Buddhists that the Buddha did it, and so in Buddhism we have the healing." "Well, can you heal the physical self?" He said, "Not yet." And so he said, "What do you mean by 'not yet'?". He said, "Oh, we monks are very busy, giving (ah) discourses and lectures and preaching so that the mind can be attuned for the spiritual level. And we want to better the mind first before we touch the physical." "And then how are you going to get the physical training?" He said, "That will come. We have not given up, although we do not have it yet. And therefore the Zen prayers in our chanting of the Sutras are very necessary in our faith, [it] is stronger than ever and we have not lost it, and someday, during our various meditations, that we shall receive that great light and then we shall know. Then we know we are ready, but don't at the present. We are striving for it, but we know we are not there. But before our meditation ends and before I go into transition I am sure it will be all enlightened and I will be able to do it."

And he said, "Thank you very much." He said, "May I come in and stay here and study all the Sutras that you have? And also I would like to hear your lectures on Buddhism because I was a Christian minister and I have faith in the Christian Bible and I've looked all over and yet I could not find any formula of healing - though I believe that Christ did it, and I still believe it." And so the monk said, "Come in." And he said "I would like to join your monks, your priests and then study here."

It took him about three years to go all through the Sutras in the temple. And when meditation hour came Dr. Usui sat with the other monks in hours and hours of meditation. And then it became very vivid to him that this was not enough, so he told the monks, "Thank you very much for your very good help and for keeping me here, and I shall like to stay on and I would like to further my studies." And the monk said, "You are most welcome, because we believe in what you are searching [for] - we believe too! And the only thing that we are doing is - besides prayer - we meditate a lot to receive that. But, if you want to further your studies, you just do it, right here in this temple."

So he said [to himself] "the Japanese character that is written in the Sutras, all these characters, originally these came from China. We have adopted the Chinese characters as Japanese characters, and so (like) when you read the Sutras, you cannot understand, but it's just like English people reading Latin. You know it, but the characters are read as written." He could do it. So finally he went very deep into the Chinese characters and became a master of the Chinese characters. And after that was completed, he said, "Not enough." He said, "After all, Buddha was a Hindu, and therefore" he said "I should study the Sanskrit. And if I study the Sanskrit, there may be something in Sanskrit, taking notes by the Buddha's disciples, because Buddha had many, many disciples, and that's how the scriptures were written."

And so, when he went into studying the Sanskrit, and when he later studied very hard to master it, he found a formula. Just as plain as mathematics. Nothing hard, but very simple. Like two and two equals four, three and three equals six, as simple as that! And so he said, "Very well,(he says) I've found it. But now, I have to try to interpret this, because it was written 2500 years ago – ancient! Because I don't know if this will work or not. But I have to go through the test. And going through this test," he said, "I cannot guarantee myself whether I will live through it, or not. But if I don't try the test," he said," everything will be lost. We'll go back to zero." And so he talked it over with the monk, and the monk said, "Yes, you are a very courageous man. Where are you going to test this, right in this temple?" He said, "No. I would like to go up into the mountains," and this was in Kyoto also.

He went up to Mount Kurma yama. And he said "I will

test myself for twenty-one days. And if I do not come back on the night of the twenty-first day, on the twenty-second day morning, send out a searching party into the forest to find my body. I will be dead." And so, with that farewell, he left, and he said "I shall go on three weeks meditation without food - only water. So he took some water up and he climbed up in the mountains where he found a stream that was close to water, and therefore he sat under a big pine tree and he started his meditation. But before he sat down, he had no timepiece, no watch, no calendar, and so how was he going to know twenty one days? So he gathered twenty one small rocks or stones and then piled it in front of him. And then his water jug and he knew where to get more water if this ran out.

There he started his meditation, and so he said, "This is the first day." And then he threw one rock away. And that's how he counted his days. And he said he expected some kind of a phenomena but he didn't know what. He didn't know what to expect. And all this time Dr. Usui , very faithfully, he read the scriptures, chanted, meditated, and then he only drank the water. And then every day came, then another day. Finally came the morning of the twenty-first, that was early morning. And he said "The darkest of night is in the earliest of morn, before sunrise is the darkest." That's how he did this. There was not even one star, no moon or any kind of a light. He said the sky was dark, just as dark as it could be. And when he finished his meditation and he said he opened his eyes and looked into the dark sky, and all he was thinking was, "This is my last meditation.".

And then he saw a flicker of light only large as a candle light, in the dark sky. And then he said, "Oh! Now, this phenomenon is very strange, but," he said, "it is happening, and I am not going to even shut my eyes, or, I shall open my eyes as wide as I can, and to witness what happens to that light." And the light began to move very fast towards him. Then he said, "Oh, the light! Now I have a chance to shirk the light, or dodge. What shall I do?" Then he said, "Even if the light strikes me, and if I fall (I don't know), or if the impact is so severe that I might drop back, or I might burn." He said," this is the test" he said" I am not going to run away, I'm going to face it." And when he faced it, he began to brace himself more (you know), and to say that: "Come! If this is it come and hit me, I am ready."

And with that, he relaxed and, his eyes wide open, he saw the light strike in the center of his forehead and naturally he said,"I made a contact he said. He fell backward because the force was so great! But then he said, "I died, because I had no sense, no feeling, my eyes just..., and my eyes were open but I couldn't see." And then he said, "I don't know how long, how many minutes I was down, but" he said," when I looked," he said "that light was gone but I could see it was beginning to have daylight and far away I could hear the roosters crowing. And far away I could see that there were movements and then I know there was going to be dawn pretty soon."

Then he happened to look a little on the right side and then he saw from the right side of his face, millions and millions of bubbles all came out, bubbling up, bubbling up, bubbling up, bubbling up, millions and millions and millions of bubbles! And these bubbles all had colors. And they had the colors of the rainbow. And he said they danced in front of him and then they went to the left and when that went he saw another streak of light - this time he says "the color of another rainbow," he said "the blue came out, and then went through the right, to the left" and then he said "the lavender came out," and then he said "some rose came out, and then the yellow came out," and he said he was counting those colors, and it had the Seven Colors, all seven And so Dr. Usui said, "Whaa! This is a phenomena! I was blessed today."

Then last of all, he saw the great white light come from the right, and then like a screen they just stood right in front of him, like a screen. And when he glued his eyes to the screen, he said, what he had studied in the Sanskrit, what he saw and studied in the Sanskrit, he said, one by one flew out, and then in golden letters, he said they just radiated out in front of him as if to say, "Remember! Remember!" And so, he said, he didn't even blink his eyes but he just studied and studied and he said, "Yes!" He said.

Then this one went to the left, (and) another came out. And all what he had studied and learned out of the Sanskrit moved in front of him as if to say, "This is it, this is it. Remember! Remember!" And so he just glued his eyes. And he said he felt no pain, no hardship, and he said he felt no hunger, no pain. He said, "I began to feel my body would float." And so in all this phenomena had passed on, and he said, "I must close my eyes and for the last meditation and he did." And he could see all the glowing letters in front of him. And so he said, "Now, I can open my eyes and throw away the last stone." And he said, "I'm going to stand up." And he stood up.

When he stood up and tried to place his feet on the ground, and he said, "They are strong. I fasted for twenty-one days but, he said, I feel I can walk back to Kyoto." Which was - in Japanese [units of distance], seventeen miles is almost about twenty five miles. "But I will reach there before sundown." And he found that [it was] as if his body had a big dinner last night. And he said that his stomach, he said, "Well, that is the first miracle, I'm not hungry. And I feel very light." Then he dusted all the pine cones and the dust and stuff. Then he picked up his cane and his straw hat and he went down the mountain.

When he went down the mountain (and) almost to the foot of the mountain. Well, he stumbled on a little rock and then lifted his toenail. The blood began to spurt out, and he felt pain. Then he said, just like anybody else would, "Ah, I hurt myself." And he took his right hand, and he held the toe. And when he felt the toe, he felt some beating "thump, thump, thump, thump" as if there was a heartbeat. Then he kept on holding it, then he said the pain began to go away. And then the blood stopped flowing. And so he said okay, two hands and he held it with two hands. And then when all the pulsation was gone, and all the pain was gone, then he saw that the blood had all dried up, but the toe had gone back to its normal position, but he could see where all the blood had come out. Then he said, "That is the second miracle".

"Now," he said "I must look for a snack bar." And when he looked around there was a bench with wool blankets and an ashtray, [a] Japanese ashtray is a big box, with pipes on the bench; you have pipes, that's all. And when you see that, in any strange place or in any park, that means 'welcome'; wool blanket is a welcome: "Please sit here. There is a snack bar close by." And so he set his cane and his straw hat and he sat down and then he looked around, he looked around. And in the right hand corner he found that there was a snack bar, and a very old man. He had an apron on, unshaved, starting the charcoal stove, you know, like the Japanese hibachi. So he walked up to him and he said, "Good morning, old man." And the man said, "Good morning, my dear monk."

He said "you are early." He said, "Yes. I would like to have that box of rice, with Japanese leftover rice in a bamboo box made, you know. And then they put the rice in there and a cover there like that rice box. If you have any leftover rice from last night, I would like to have that rice, and as soon as you make the tea, I would like to have that piece of nori that you made today. I would like to have that nori and also some (ah) salted cabbage and also (ah) dried fish if you have any." (That's a regular Japanese breakfast.) And he said, "I shall wait for you at the bench." And so the old gentleman said, "I would love you to have the rice but you have to wait until I make soft rice gruel, like mush."

He said, "According to your dedication," (that means Dr. Usui was dedicated to be[ing] there) "many people go up this mountain, this is known as a very famous mountain for meditation. And when they come down in seven days, one week of meditation, the beard is much shorter, and then some do two weeks, but according to your dedication you've been up there three weeks. And when you do not eat for twenty one days," he say "I cannot let you have that rice, and that hot tea and all those things to go with [them] because you're going to have acute indigestion, and when you have that," he says, " I have no medicine, and I cannot help you. And therefore, since it is seventeen miles away in the city of Kyoto, there are doctors. But I cannot reach the doctor. So therefore" (he says)" you have to wait." So Dr. Usui said, "Thank you, you are very kind. But I think I shall try it." So he crawled to the table, and went for that rice pot. He carried it, because he didn't want the old man to take away. And left it by his wood bench. And he waited, and in a few minutes the old man gave up already, He said, "Well, if he wants to do it his way, fine."

He sent the girl, it was his granddaughter, about fifteen years old, and she brought out the tray with the rice bowl, chopsticks, and hot tea, pot of hot tea and with all the other ingredients to go with the rice. And so she put this on the wood bench. But this girl was crying - tears running down, and not only that - her face was swollen. And she had a big towel here, tied up here like rabbit ears. And so Dr. Usui looked at her and said, "My dear young girl, (he said) why do you cry?" She said, "Oh, my dear monk, three days and three nights I have a toothache so bad that I cannot stop my tears. And I cannot eat. I didn't have any kind of a food for three days and three nights. And it hurts so much I cannot stop my tears. And yet the dentist is so far away, I cannot ask my grandfather to take me seventeen miles to Kyoto. And therefore I have to just suffer and cry. But I can't stop my tears."

So Dr. Usui stood up and began to dig into her cheek and said, "Is this the one? Is this the one?" Then when he came to the right one she said "Yes, yes, yes." "Oh, all right!". Then he put his hand there. And then the girl began to blink, blink the eyes, and she said, "My dear monk, you have just made magic!" He said, "How do you feel now?" She said, "The toothache is gone!". "Is it really? Are you telling me the truth?" She said: "Yes, I do not have to shed tears any more. I can stop crying." And then she took off the rabbit ears and wiped her face. And by that time Dr. Usui put two hands on. And then he said, "Now, I think you are well." And the girl smiled, thanked him, and went to the grandfather. And she said, "Grandfather, I took off my rabbit ears, the toothache is gone. And he is no ordinary monk, he makes magic!" That's what the girl said.

So the grandfather came out, wiping his hands on the apron, and he said, "My dear monk, you did us a great service. You just did magic on my granddaughter, stopped the toothache. We are so grateful, oh we are so grateful! Because she was suffering. And for our gratitude," he said, "the food is on the house. And this is all we can offer, because we do not have much, you know." And Dr. Usui put his hands together and said, "Thank you! I accept your gratitude. Thank you very much!" And he said, "All right, now, for my food!" And he stirred the rice bowl, and then put the hot tea and started shoveling with the chopsticks. And he ate happily, so the people didn't disturb him while he ate. But they were wishing that he wouldn't have any kind of indigestion.

Dr. Usui enjoyed his breakfast this way, and he said, "Now,(he said) this is the fourth miracle. The third miracle was the toothache gone." And he said, "I have no indigestion." He said, "Now, I'm ready to start on my seventeen mile hike and by sundown I shall reach the temple according to schedule." And he did. And when he did, he knocked at the doorbell, and that little page boy came out. And he said, "Dr. Usui , we are so happy that you are home, because if you did not come home tonight, you know we were going to send a searching party tomorrow morning as you requested." You see, all these little monks in the temple, they are about six to ten years old. They go in when they are six years old to study Buddhism. And they are very witty and very smart, you see, but that's how he tried to tease him.

And he said, first thing Dr. Usui said, "How is our dear monk?" "Oh, he's suffering from arthritis and backache, and this is a cool evening, so he is hugging the chapel stove, and he is under silk covers." This is what the little page boy said. "So if you go and take a bath, and while you do this, we'll lay out your clean clothes and warm up your food. And after you've eaten your dinner, then you will visit the monk, who will be waiting for you. And he will be very happy to know that you are home and I shall deliver that message. So, go take your bath." And so he did.

After his dinner, he went to see the monk. And the monk was sure in bed, hugging the chapel stove. He said, "My dear monk, I am back." The first thing he asked was "How was it? How was your meditation?"."Success." That is the only word he could use, was 'success'. And the monk said, "Oh, I feel so happy, I feel so happy," he said, "Let me hear about it." And so he said, "Yes, and while I talk to you, (he said) I would like to put my hands on top of the silk covers," where he had the silk futon covers on him. And then told him all about what had happened, and from the time he sat for meditation and on the twenty-first morning, and what has happened throughout the day. And then it was late at night already when he said, "Very good, very good, we shall hear more about it, and let me think tonight, "the monk said. "And by the way, my pain is all gone. I can sleep now. I can leave the stove alone, my body feels wonderful! I feel that I am very full of energy," and so he said, "this is what you call Reiki.' He said "Yes, Reiki.". "So... we'll talk more about it tomorrow morning after our breakfast."

Dr. Usui had a good night's sleep, and so the monks next morning after breakfast, first thing Dr. Usui said, "What shall I do to experiment with this?" And so they talked over and over and other monks came in, and they decided that the best place for him to experiment was to try and go into one of the very big slums in Kyoto. And so they chose one of the largest slums, and in the slum they found all kinds of diseases, even leprosy.

He went there as a monk, dressed up like a monk, but as a vegetable peddler. So he had one basket of vegetables in the front, and one in the back, and then he had a pole, and he carried that. And he walked and went into the slum, and all the beggars came out. And he said, "Oh, we are having a different kind of a guest today!" And so Dr. Usui said, "Please, I would like to be one of you; I would like to live here." And so, they looked at him and said, "If you want to stay here, we have a chief. And so we shall call him." So like in any gypsy camp you find a gypsy chief, you know, of the clan. And in this slum there was also a chief. So, when this chief was there, he came and he said, "I understand that you want to live here and become one of us." He said, "Yes." "He said, "If that is the case, all right, let me have the vegetables." And he took all the vegetables. And he said, "No need to wear new clothes here." He said, " Bring the initiation clothes."

And so they brought the rags, dirty, smelly rags. And then took off all his clothes, and when they undressed him, they found a money belt on him - money belt, and also the chief smiled, and he said. "You see, my eyes are really sharp and keen" he said. "I could see all through those shining new clothes, new skirt, new kimono, and a cloak you know. I could see the money belt. And that has to be released." And so he released it and so the chief took it. Then he said, "All right, bring the clothes. And put on the initiation clothes." And he said, "All right, now obi - and put the obi around." Then he said, "Now, you have gone through the initiation and you can stay here. But what are you going to do?"

He said, "I will not beg for food outside of this compound. I would like you to give me a cottage by myself where you can send patients and I am going to heal." "Very good, that's a wonderful exchange for food. All right, we will feed you three meals a day, and give you a place to stay and where all the sick people visit you. We need it. And we have all kinds: impetigo, we have all kinds of diseases, even tuberculosis and leprosy. You're not afraid to touch them?" He said,"No, I am a healer", he said. So, I shall work from sunup to sundown, and therefore I want my meals brought up here. This is a very, very good thing." So this pleased the slum chief very much, and of course they took all the money and everybody divided the vegetables and stuff, and that was fine.

Dr. Usui started the next morning, and he started to do it. But before he started, he chose his clients. All the ones that were sick got in a group, and then he chose young people, because he felt if they are young, the cause must be shallow. So he started to work on the cause and effect, cause and effect. And he was right! The older the person and the deeper the disease, he found it took many days and months. And so, when he worked on the shallow cases, in about a week they were all better and ready for a new life. So he said "You go to this address." And this was the temple, the Zen temple. "And ask for this monk and he will give you a new name and he will give you a job. And you go into the city or anywhere they assign you, and become an honest citizen and forget the slum. Now that we have helped you physically, you are a complete whole." You see? And so this went on for years.

Dr. Usui had lots and lots of experiences. So, to make a long story short, if you ask me, was he successful? Was he a success? Far from it! Because Dr. Usui when he left Kyoto and his ministry, he left in search of how to heal the physical. He thought he was a very good minister, so when he came back and went all the way to the temple, searching, there all the monks said, "Spiritual first, the mind first and physical second. So why should we bother with the human body when we have medicine and doctors?" So Dr. Usui was disappointed, because that was not his aim. His aim was to do something for the body. So he forgot the spiritual side. And then all these people went out of the slum. They weren't easy - he was there seven years.

One evening twilight he found himself at the Dejo. So he walked around the compound to see how much accomplishment. Then he found a familiar face. He said, "I don't know your name but your face looks familiar." And he said, "You too, and you too!" "But I don't know your name. Who are you?" He said, "Oh, you should remember. I was one of the first guys that came here and got healed, and then you sent us to the temple. And when you sent us to the temple they gave us a new name, and we had a new job, and so we became honorable citizens and then we worked."

(And) so Dr. Usui was disappointed, he received the greatest shock of his life. And he just threw himself on the ground, and there was a mud puddle, but he didn't, he had no choice, he just threw himself. And he said he cried and cried like a little child, and he said, "Oh, what did I do?" He said: "I did not save a Soul. So the physical is number two and the spiritual is number one. Therefore, all the churches in Kyoto were right!

They were right and I was wrong. And therefore I am going to heal, absolutely heal! No beggars, no more beggars, no more beggars. And it was my fault for making them come back here as beggars."

He blamed himself, he said. "So while his head was in the mud puddle, he began to think and he said, "I forgot to teach them before they left - gratitude. All you beggars are here because they are people only greedy, greedy. Greed, greed. Want, want - nothing to return, and nothing to show gratitude." So, therefore, the five ideals were born at that time. And the ideals are: Just for today, do not anger; just for today, do not worry; number three, we shall count our blessings and honor our fathers and mothers, and our teachers and neighbors; and honor our food; we shall not waste any food, because food is also God-given, although the farmers they do cultivate it. But if you do have famine, you do not have food. But we just have to show gratitude towards food. And then, number four, make an honest living. We have to work in order to make an honest living, this is number four. And number five is to be kind to everything that has life.

These are the five ideals of Reiki; it was born at that instant when Dr. Usui recognized his failure. And so he said, "If I had taught them the spiritual side of it first, and then healed the body," he said, "It would have been effective." But now all his patients were coming back. He said, "How many years did you work outside?" "A couple years." "How many years did you work?" "Only about a year and a half. But it's easier to fill up my stomach rather than work," he said. "Begging is a very easy profession. And (he said) I fill up my stomach better than working and hustling by myself." And therefore he said, "Beggars are beggars - no more Reiki. No more healing." And that is when Dr. Usui walked out of the compound.

Then he made a pilgrimage all over Japan, you know the main island part from the north to the south on foot. And he chose a big mall, where the people will be there. And he took a torch, and lighted the torch and he would be walking up and down the mall where there were thousands of people. So, one young man would come to him, and he said, "My dear monk, if you are looking for light," he said, "You don't need that torch. Today we have a lot of sunshine. This is a beautiful day," he said. "You don't need this torch light."

He said, "We can see." He said, "Yes, that is very true. But, I am looking and searching for people that have very sad, depressed minds. People are unhappy. I am searching for people that need this light to brighten their hearts and to take away their depression, and cleansing their character and their mind and body. And so, if you want to hear this lecture, come to the church." And so he visited every temple this way, on foot. And into one of his favorite suguoka you know, in one part of Japan, that's when he met Chujiro Hayashi, he was a retired Naval reserve. And he was a commander in the Navy. And when he heard Dr. Usui speak this way, he got interested, and so he attended his lecture.

When he attended his lecture, Dr. Usui kind of pointed him out after the lecture, and he said, "I see that you are a man (ah) that is a leader." He said, "Yes, I am. I have just served my time as a navy commander in the Imperial Majesty's force. And now, I am reserve in the navy, so I have earned all that." So he said, "But you are too young to retire. So why do you not join me in this crusade, and then to help people? I think you would be a very good person to do this." And so Dr. Hayashi said, "Well, I will try. If you recommend so," he said, "I am interested too." And at that time, Dr. Hayashi was only forty-five. And so he walked with Dr. Usui all over. He said that he was with him, I don't know, I forgot how many years, but until Dr. Usui died, went into transition, and when he did, and he said I need to go and Dr. Usui announced that it was Dr. Chujiro Hayashi that was going to pursue this Usui System in the art of healing.

This is the life story of Dr. Usui , which I have heard from Dr. Hayashi. And during his reign Dr. Hayashi never changed the system. It is even until today, and even my students, and my followers, learned this art of healing at the Usui Reiki Ryoho and in English, the suffix is Japanese, but it is the Usui System in the Art of Healing. And this word 'Reiki' is [a] Japanese word, but in English it is 'Universal Life Energy'. But I use it as Reiki because I learned in Japan, and therefore I still continue to say it in the short word 'Reiki'.

Dr. Usui had this experience at the beggar's camp. And when he was down in the mud, his body in the hole - that's when his thinking came out and he said, "Ah! I have made a great mistake." He said. "All the churches were right - spiritual first. And here (he said), I did not preach the spiritual side, but I was so interested in healing the body that I just thought the best thing was to do the healing to make them well enough to appreciate, so that they could go out into the world as normal people." But he failed. And when he failed, these five ideals were born. And in these five ideals, where did the beggars fail?

The beggars have no sense of gratitude. And therefore, he said, "I'll heal it! No more free treatments! No more Reiki, Reiki, Reiki, or classes, because they will never learn to appreciate." And this is very true, that Dr. Usui forgot at that moment he was so happy that he could do it. And so he said, "The seven years of experience, I shall charge it to bad experiences which I could not master. "Therefore," he said, "no more Reiki - free, free." He said. "Everything has to be on the upper-upper, so that we will have a good mind, and a good body, good mind and body to make a human being a complete whole."

And this is very, very true. Because in 1936, when I came back from Japan, and Dr. Hayashi had warned me. He had warned me, he had said, "Whenever you become a master, never do it free because they will never use it, because it was free. Because it was free, it has no value." But once again, I asked my teacher: "Dr. Hayashi," I said, "will you permit and consent that I have one class free? And that is for all the people that have helped me through this year of sorrow and my sickness." I said, "I would like to teach them and give them a free lesson in Reiki so that they could benefit." So Dr. Hayashi said, "Now that you are well, you can return your gratitude by giving them treatment when needed, but not to say I'll hold a class for you people, and then to use it, and then to benefit yourself because," he said, "that will never be acceptable." Now with that understanding, I said to myself, "Well, I have to try."

The first people that I gave free lessons [to] were my best friend and relatives. They were my in-laws. All my in-laws had free lessons, and then all my neighbors, they had free lessons. And then when my two sisters came, I said "Wait, wait." I said. "I'm not going to teach you yet." So, my sisters were kind of upset, and said, "Well, we heard here from all your neighbors and all the in-laws that you taught them something really wonderful." But I said, "I have to see their success too." So I said, "At this moment, I will say no for the moment." Then I waited.

One day I was hanging my laundry, and then the neighbor came and said, "My daughter didn't go to school today, because she had a little stomach ache. And so I brought her. I said, "Why don't you go in and give her a treatment?" So, I said, "Why? Why did I teach you? Why don't you try? You don't even try!!". She said, "No. Why should I? You're the expert here that lives next to me. So, it's easier to bring her to you than do it myself because I know she'll get well." And so that was one disappointment. And then on the other side of the town, another one said, "Oh, my daughter has runny nose and the teacher said 'go home because it's contagious, she has the flu.' And so I brought my daughter, I want you to give her a treatment." I said, "Didn't I teach you?"

She said, "Yes. Well, why should I, when I have a car and can run to you? You're the expert here, and when you do it I know they are going to get well." And so I said, "You never even tried to use it?" She said, "No, why should I?" You see? No gratitude whatever! And believe it or not, I hid in my house and I cried. And then I looked towards Japan, and bowed my head to Dr. Hayashi, and also towards Dr. Usui 's grave. And I said, "Forgive me for being wrong. I did not help any person because they did not accept this gratefully and spiritually, because they didn't spend a penny." And so I said, "It is very sad, but I will turn them down hereafter, so that I will make them use it."

Then after three months my sisters came again. And they said, "Now, do you have time?" I said "Yes, I have time. But do you really want to learn Reiki?" And so my sisters said, "Yes, we heard good things about you, but what is it, that all your in-laws know Reiki, and [why] not your own flesh and blood?" "Because there is a fee." "Oh, there is a fee. How much?" I said, "Three hundred dollars." And so she said, "Well, I don't have that kind of money right now. So I have to go home and ask my husband." I said, "Very good. And you don't have to pay me cash [all at] one time, but (I said) you can pay in installments. But I will not go to your house to collect the money. Every payday you come [to] my house."

So, my sister was in a little... not so happy, happily ...; she went home, she talked over with her husband, and she said her husband said, "Did you ask your sister that you would like to learn Reiki?" And my sister said to her husband, "Yes." "Well, if you had asked her that you want to learn Reiki," he said, "[then] you pay the fee. And ask her; you will pay her by installments. And if she says she is not coming here to collect the money, you take the money to her, which is proper. That is proper, everything is proper. And so you'd better do it and that is my answer." That's what he said. Because he said it was okay, my sister came back and then she said, "Yes, we will pay you in installments, $25 a month," she said. "Fine, fine. I'll help you. Just leave , that's all."

My two sisters learned, and they paid me in installments. I didn't feel really very happy about this, but it was the principle that I had to follow. And then what happened, the first time her daughter had asthma, she said, because she had paid such a big price, she had to use it. "I couldn't take her to the doctor. You know, sister, it worked! And I am happy, I learned, and it worked. And she will sleep better again and Good" So, I said, "Now you get your lessons?"

She said, "Yes," she said. "I came to apologize, you know, for not being happy-happy and being radiant over it, until I experienced it. But I know why you charged me. I know.

Because you wanted me to be good, and a good practitioner, and then I do not have any more medicine bills and doctor bills, I don't have to go to the hospital every time she has a cold, or every time she is asthmatic, or every time bronchitis or a stomach ache." And she said, "You know, I have three children. And so," she said, " now I understand why, and here today, I hang my head down very low, and then I come to thank you and I appreciate it so much, I'll make good use of it." And she did!.

Today she is a very successful woman. She has not failed in her business. She has her own business. And then she's a great healer, yes. And then she said that "Everlasting I have this power, everlasting. It was the cheapest investment rather than buy a car." She said. "Couldn't be any cheaper than this!" she said. And every time she sees me she says, "I give you Reiki." She gives me treatments all the time...every day if I am with her. You see? And that is the gratitude.

And all today when I have seen these twenty-four people that I have given the free lessons, not one of them are successful. Not even in business or in their health. And therefore, my teachers were right, they were absolutely right.

[End of tape]

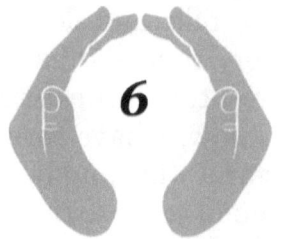

6   *Analyzing the facts*

W.L Rand says that, Speculation based on knowledge of other ancient healing systems has led to a plausible hypothesis that may shed some light on the pre-Usui origins of Reiki. There is a Tibetan Buddhist healing technique called the Medicine Buddha. It involves the laying-on of hands similar to Reiki. The ability to do Medicine Buddha healing is transmitted to the student through an empowerment given by the teacher similar to a Reiki attunement. There are other spiritual lineages in Tibetan Buddhism involving the transmission of ability or value through empowerments. Since Tibetan Buddhism is the only form of Buddhism that uses empowerments, it is likely that the Reiki Dr. Usui rediscovered was formerly a Tibetan technique that had been lost.

It is known that a spiritual lineage of this type may stop due to the failure of the teacher to pass it on. The lineage may then resume hundreds or thousands of years later when a monk or spiritual seeker receives instruction and empowerment during a mystical experience. Perhaps this is what happened to Dr. Usui. Perhaps he had been a Reiki Master in a past life and this gave him the determination to seek the healing power again. Perhaps the lineage had come to an end only to be started again when Dr. Usui's Reiki was reactivated during his mystical experience.

There is also a different story about the Buddhist origins of Reiki according to the followers of Medicine Dharma Reiki. Their version is, Dr. Usui created or formulated a system of secular healing and simple spiritual practice. This he formulated for anyone of any faith or no faith, yet the origin of the system was Buddhism. The Buddhist material he taught only to Buddhists, those who had taken Refuge in Mahayana or Vajrayana Buddhism, and had the commitment to practice its teachings. According to Dr. Usui there were 7 levels of advanced studies, these do not relate to the 7 levels of Radiance Technique, or any other "invented" or channeled system of "additional Reiki".

We could say the foundation was the outer teachings, which constitutes Reiki degrees 1-3. The advanced levels were the inner Buddhist teachings relating to the sacred Tantra which he had studied and expounded together with other related Buddhist teachings from the esoteric school of Buddhism in Japan. The material Dr. Usui studied relating to Reiki came from the Buddha in Northern India, via China to Japan. These teachings had arrived in Japan in the 8th & 9th centuries mostly transmitted by Kobo Daishi (Kukai). (Note: Buddhism was just establishing in Tibet at this time). One of the Tantras that Usui taught was known as the "Tantra of the Lightning Flash". It appears as the centuries past, this Tantra fell into disuse, only to be found again by the physician Mikao Usui at the turn of the 19th Century.

As he researched this in Japan, he found parallel teachings coming from Tibet. Dr. Usui brought forth or actualized the Buddhist teachings of the Tantra of the Lightning Flash and other Dharma (Buddhist teachings) because there was not a living lineage of teachers practicing its teachings. He taught this material, but again its spiritual aspect (the inner Buddhist teachings) fell into disuse after Usui's death in 1926. Fortunately, the written teachings of Usui were retrieved from obscurity in Japan in 1946, during the liberation after World War 2, in a lacquered casket which was bought from an itinerant monk seeking money to rebuild his monastery in north-eastern Tokyo and feed his fellow monks.

In 1962 the contents were appraised by the British Museum, this revealed writings from the 11th Century through to the 1920's. The title pages were translated, and they included copies of the Mahavairocana Sutra, copies of commentaries and lectures by Kukai and other Shingon teachers; a 13th Century

Tendai document which included excerpts from several Buddhist Sutras (including the Lotus and Flower Adornment Sutra); a collection of medical and healing teachings revealed by Sakyamuni Buddha called "The Tantra of the Lightning Flash"; numerous letters and notes written by Dr Usui and his student Dr. Watanabe. Usui developed the healing system from Esoteric Buddhism in the early 1900's, one of his successors; Seiji Takamori researched the Tibetan Buddhist connection.

Venerable Seiji Takamori, was a Japanese Zen Buddhist monk and a Reiki Master who traveled to Northern India, Nepal & Tibet in search of enlightenment. There he studied for 20 years and found spiritual practices which contained (in another form) all he had previously learned in Reiki (but there was a lot more). Thus, he concluded, this was a parallel line of teaching from the Buddha related to healing and meditation.

The essence of Ven. Seiji Takamori's discovery is taught from his Usui Reiki lineage, now called Reiki Jin-Kei Do (The Way of Compassion & Wisdom through Reiki), and the advanced Buddhist practices as Buddho-EnerSense. The Buddha was known as "The Great Physician" and his teachings are the medicine to alleviate all suffering in samara (the cycle of birth and death). To think of healing on a physical level, or of this lifetime, is to take a very narrow view of healing. That said, Usui took the complex teachings of Buddhism and simplified them so that anyone could have access to its supportive and healing qualities at a certain level. Dr. Usui was following the paradigm of both Jesus and Sakyamuni, in that, acting from the heart of compassion, he tried to relate his teachings in accordance to the student's ability, and as they developed in their practice and understanding they were taught more.

Recently there had so many researches about the origins, which is mainly done by Frank Arjava Petter, W.L Rand, Dave King & Melissa Riggall and Lawerence Ellyard. There are also many internet sites which had conducted research. From this entire source we can assume history. Most Reiki teachers simply accepted Mrs. Takata's story as being factual until the research which was mainly done by Frank Arjava Petter and mentioned in his book, Reiki Fire. With the help of his Japanese wife, Chetna and Shizuko Akimoto, a Japanese Reiki master, Arjava contacted a number of important sources of information concerning the history of Reiki. Included were several people who learned Reiki from some of Usui 's early teachers, namely a Mr. Oishi and a Mr. Fumio Ogawa.

Arjava also spoke to members of Usui 's family and members of the Usui Shiki Reiki Ryoho, which is the original Reiki organization started by Usui in Tokyo. From these contacts he filled in some missing information on the history of Reiki and discovered other valuable facts. This information provides more accurate insight into who Usui was, what motivated him to rediscover Reiki and how he and his students practiced.

In the original Reiki story, Mikao Usui is portrayed as a Christian, teaching theology at the Doshisha Christian University in Japan. However, derived from Usui 's personal notes translated by lama Yeshe, describes him as a devoted Shingon Buddhist. Usui never taught at Doshisha University and was never a Principal of any school. Usui was also very skeptical about the Christian doctrine, although he later befriended a Christian physician, who became a mentor for Dr. Usui with his medical training. This is also described in subsequent chapters of Usui 's manuscripts published by lama Yeshe.

Today, Usui's wife's cousin states that he was a Tendai lay monk and we know that his ashes are buried in a Pure Land Buddhist graveyard (where his memorial stone stands) and also no evidence to suggest that he was specifically a Zen monk, though today it is understood that he definitely was Buddhist (either Tendai or Pure Land).

In Mrs. Takata's story, Dr. Usui is also said to have traveled to the United States to receive his Doctorate in Medicine from the University of Chicago in the late1880s. There are variations of this western story some masters says that he was never a doctor and instead studied theology in the United States.

Recent research has clearly shows that Dr. Mikao Usui never traveled outside Japan's sacred islands, except on two Occasions, once to China where he studied Chinese Herbal Medicine and once to Hokkaido (Japan's northern island), where he had a short and somewhat arduous Journey. Dr. Usui later tells this story in the following chapter of manuscripts published by lama Yeshe. In the Usui Memorial it is written that Dr. Usui traveled extensively to some countries. It is not mentioned in his journals about these journeys.

Indeed, if Dr. Usui had traveled to the United States and had studied medicine in the 1880s then Medical Faculty of Chicago University will mention his name but the astonishing thing is Chicago University had not yet been established during that period. It wasn't until the 1890s that the Medical Faculty began in the city of Chicago established which was after ten years regarding Usui meant to have studied there!. This has been researched in the US and no documentation of a person called Mikao Usui from that period can be found in their database.

According to Lawerence Ellyard, Usui was a Medical Physician and had received his training from Western physicians in the 1880s, some of which were Christians who were sent to Japan with the first missionaries. The Chicago link, where perhaps Mrs. Takata introduced the theme, comes from one of Dr. Usui 's friend, a Medical Doctor who he met in 1916. Usui 's western friend had received his training from the then established Chicago Medical faculty. Other aspects of Mrs. Takata's story describe Dr. Usui carrying a flaming torch when he visited villages, as a symbol of the light teachings' he was offering. This story however, describes the great Buddhist master Kobo Daishi who was responsible for founding Shingon Buddhism in Japan.

The torch bearer, Kobo Daishi used this symbol as his calling card; he would carry a flaming torch during the day and was responsible for bringing Buddhism to Japan, not an easy undertaking. Kobo Daishi also brought with him the 'Tantra of the Lightning Flash', the essential teachings of what became known as Reiki.

According to literature at the Mt. Kurama temple, in 770 A.D. a priest named Gantei climbed Mount Kurama, led by a white horse. His soul was enlightened with the realization of Bishamonten, the protector of the northern quarter of the Buddhist heaven and the spirit of the sun. Gantei founded the Buddhist temple on Mt. Kurama, which went through many stages of development and restoration and now contains many temples and pagodas. The temple was formerly part of the Tendai sect of Buddhism. Since 1949, it has been part of the newly founded Kurama-Kokyo sect of Buddhism.

Many variations of the western Reiki story also describe Dr. Usui 's experience on Mt. Kurama Yama. But one thing is certain Usui received empowerments or enlightenment (Satotri) from this holy mountain during his 21 days of meditation. According to manuscripts "These spheres manifested before me like bubbles rising on water and then I became aware of their importance and the methodology with which to employ them... (They) sank into me and bestowed upon me the power to impart this healing modality to everyone". He had visited the sacred mountain many times from his childhood itself, to contemplate and regularly enjoyed visiting this sacred place.

According to Rand, Usui's personal and business life was failing. As a sensitive spiritualist, Usui had spent much time meditating at power spots on Mt. Kurama where he had received his early Buddhist training. So he decided to travel to this holy mountain, where he enrolled in Isyu Guo, a twenty-one-day training course sponsored by the Tendai Buddhist Temple located there. We do not know for certain what he was required to do during this training, but it is likely that fasting, meditation, chanting and prayers were part of the practice.

In addition, we know there is a small waterfall on Mt. Kurama where even today people go to meditate. This meditation include standing under the waterfall and allowing the waters to strike and flow over the top of the head, a practice which is said to activate the crown chakra. Japanese Reiki Masters think that Usui may have used this meditation as part of his practice. In any case, it was during the Isyu Guo training that the great Reiki energy entered his crown chakra. This greatly enhanced his healing abilities and he realized he had received a wonderful new gift - the ability to give healing to others without depleting his own energy!

Other information received from Shizuko Akimoto is that Usui studied many things before rediscovering Reiki. He took what he studied and combined what seemed right into the Usui system of healing. This is apparent in the "Reiki Ideals" which we now know came from the Meiji Emperor. This is indicated in the inscription on the Usui memorial, located at Saihoji temple. This inscription also indicates Usui studied many things, but his life was not going well when he decided to go to Mt. Kurama to meditate for answers. Perhaps he was looking for a personal transformation for which the mountain is noted and for help in healing his life. It seems he did what many of us have done when our lives have not gone well and we looked to the spiritual for answers and healing. He opened himself to the higher power and not only received a healing for him, but a way to help others.

The Usui Precepts originated with a source other than Usui . "Usui created Gokai (the 5 principles) getting hints from a book "Kenzon no Gebri" written by Dr. Suzuki Bizan (published in March, 1914.) The book says "Just for today, do not get angry, do not feel fear, be honest, work hard, and be kind to others." (From Gendai Reiki Healing Training Text)

Usui memorial stone is located at the Saihoji Temple in the Suginami district of Tokyo. The memorial was created by the Usui Shiki Reiki Ryoho shortly after Usui 's transition. This is the organization which Usui started to promote the practice and teaching of Reiki. The memorial site is maintained by the Usui Shiki Reiki Ryoho. This was verified by officials of the Saihoji Temple where the memorial is located. The memorial consists of a large monolith about four feet wide and ten feet tall. On it, written in old style Japanese kanji, is a description of Usui 's life and his discovery and use of Reiki. It is located in a public cemetery at the Saihoji Temple next to Usui 's grave stone where his ashes, along with those of his wife and son, have been placed.

The inscription on the memorial stone was written by Mr. Okata who is believed to be a member of the Usui Shiki Reiki Ryoho and Mr. Ushida, who became president after Usui died. There are many important and interesting details included in the inscription. We were surprised that the Usui Shiki Reiki Ryoho still exists because part of the "traditional" story stated that all the members of this group died in the war or had stopped using Reiki and that Mrs. Takata was the only adhering teacher of the Usui system in the world. We now know the Usui Shiki Reiki Ryoho has always existed and still exists today. They have been teaching and practicing Reiki in Japan all this time.

Shizuko Akimoto shared additional information about Usui and the history of Reiki. According to her research with Mr. Ogawa and other members of the Usui Shiki Reiki Ryoho, there was never a mandatory fee for Reiki treatments. Dr. Hayashi charged whatever people could pay and if they were poor, he treated them for free. His Reiki business was not lucrative, but was done out of a desire to help people. Many of his students received their Reiki training in return for working at his clinic. If Usui became popular helping people who suffered from the Tokyo earthquake as it states on his memorial, it is likely that he did not insist on everyone paying a fee for his treatments, but like Dr. Hayashi, must have treated many for free.

According to Arjava Petter, there is no title of "Grandmaster" or "Lineage Bearer" in the organization started by Usui . The person in charge of the organization is the president. Usui was the first president of the Usui Shiki Reiki Ryoho. Since then, there have been five successive presidents: Mr. Ushida, Mr. Taketomi, Mr. Watanabe, Mr. Wanami, and the current president, Ms. Kimiko Koyama. Dr. Hayashi was a respected teacher, but was not a president and had no other responsibilities. Mr. Hayashi was one of many respected disciples of Usui-Sensei, but not more and not less than that. In the old days disciples like Mr. Hayashi who were granted the teacher status by the president often had their own disciples. This is why there are so many different Reiki streams flowing all over Japan. However there is no question about Mr. Kondo's leadership.

There other information's from Reiki international web site they states that, the word Reiki does appear in the Reiki precepts, but the word 'Reiki' seems there to mean 'a gift of Satotri. The name 'Reiki' came later, probably introduced by the Gakkai's founders. The next revelation is that the purpose of Usui's method was to achieve Satotri, to find one's spiritual path, to heal oneself. Usui's system was not really about treating others. Treating others was not emphasized; it was not focused upon; it was a side-issue.

The vast majority of Usui's students started out as his clients, people who came to him because they wanted something treated. He would routinely give people empowerments (connect them to Reiki) so that they could treat themselves in between appointments with him, and if they wanted to take things further then they could start formal training. The training was rather like martial arts training: you had an open-ended commitment to study with Usui, not a fixed-length training course, and it was only when you had developed sufficiently that you were invited to move on to higher levels.

According to Johan Roelofse who is a Reiki Master from South Africa who has made the journey from standard Western Reiki into Japanese 'Gendai' Reiki, and beyond, The purpose of the Reiki system was complete spiritual awakening (Satotri). In the West, Reiki is often seen as a form of alternative therapy. Yes, healing was a part of the system, but spiritual development was the true purpose. As such, various Buddhist sutras and meditative practices were an integral part of the system. One of these, the Lotus Repentance meditation, is said to be the meditation Usui practiced during his 21 day retreat at Mount Kurama. It is at Mount Kurama that he experienced his full awakening, after which he developed his healing methods.

The healing side of Usui Teate also differs from what is known in Western Reiki. Usui apparently didn't use standardized hand positions, apart perhaps from treating the head. He mainly made used of Byosen (energy sensing) and Reiji (spiritual guidance) when treating people. He also didn't use both hands very often, but rather used an energy focusing technique with one hand to treat problem areas. Apart from this, various other practices, such as healing with the eyes and the breath were incorporated into his healing methods.

It is not fully palpable how Usui taught his system. What seems to be the case is that he taught a three level system, consisting of different modules. Level one (Shoden – the first teachings) was about connecting to the Reiki energy and learning to use it for healing. A variety of meditative and energy practices were also taught. Level two (Okuden – the inner teachings) was divided into two sections. In the first section the focus and harmony energies were taught as well as Byosen and Reiji.

In the second section, the connection energy and distant healing were taught. These three energies became the basis for the three-second degree symbols taught by Takata. One of the biggest surprises about Usui Teate is that Usui didn't use symbols. In fact, he taught the symbols to only three people, one being Hayashi. It is believed that he included the symbols as some kind of training wheels for individuals having difficulty connecting directly to the energy. Lieu symbols, he originally taught students to connect directly to the different energies. He also made use of meditations and sacred Shinto kotodama (seed sounds) to invoke the energies.

In the West these were replaced by saying the "names" of the symbols three times. Level three (Shinpiden – the mystery teachings) was devoted to further spiritual awakening. It also consisted of two sections, the first being for spiritual development and the second for becoming a teacher of the Usui method. Usui apparently also gave certain higher empowerments to students who have completed level 3. There is not much known about these empowerments in the West, but they likely had to do with further spiritual awakening.

At the URRI 2001 Workshop in Madrid, Spain, Mr. Hiroshi Doi explained what the Usui Reiki Ryoho Gakkai teaches as Usui 's typical way of giving a Reiki treatment. He said that Sensei would use the Reiji technique to discover the area of greatest need for healing that was required by the patient. Then he would apply Reiki there, usually with one hand. He would extend his middle and ring finger together, forwards and downwards at an angle, using them as the main focus for the energy. His index and smallest fingers were extended straight out, to act as radiators to dispel any negative energy (the thumb was up and acted this way as well).

(Note: Arjava Petter illustrated a version of this in his book The Original Handbook of Dr. Mikao Usui) In this way, Doi-sensei said, Usui would typically give 3-minute healing. A common reason for this was the belief that most ailments arise from the brain. Usui taught only treating the head, Treating around the head and finally placing most energy into the crown. (Source: Eguchi manuals). It is thus only necessary to offer energy (Qi) to the head and thorax in order to 'treat' the entire body mind.

According to Mr. Tsutomu Oishi, who learnt Reiki from one of Usui -Sensei's students: Kozo Ogawa (- a relative of Fumio Ogawa,) during the 1950's, but has not been involved with it for over thirty years. A failed business venture had left Usui-Sensei with large debts, and the experience had led him to the conclusion that there was something more to life than striving for material wealth. This realization would start him on a quest culminating in his experience on Kurama Yama, where, Tsutomu says, Usui used to regularly meditate under a waterfall (note: this is a practice common to practitioners of 'Shugendo').

According to Tsutomu, during Usui's lifetime a Reiki Centre was set up in Shizouka and was run by Kozo Ogawa, who was a talented healer. Mr. Ogawa - a retailer of school uniforms - would treat any sick children he came in contact with. Tsutomu maintained that both Kozo Ogawa and Usui used to give Reiki charged crystal balls to their students to employ in the healing process. (These balls would apparently be placed directly on the site of ailment or injury.) He says students also received a Reiki Manual. This manual included a set of treatment guidelines, as well as describing symptoms and giving an explanation of what Reiki is.

According to W.L.Rand, during his mystical experience on Mt. Kurama, Dr. Usui received the ability to do Reiki treatments, the Reiki symbols and the ability to pass Reiki on to others. Later he added the Reiki Ideals and the idea that one needs to receive compensation for a treatment. Dr. Hayashi added the standard hand positions, the three degrees and their attunement processes. Mrs. Takata added the fee structure previously mentioned. The required waiting periods between classes were added by several of Mrs. Takata's Masters after she passed on. After Mrs. Takata's transition, a few teachers began making changes in the way they taught Reiki. Most of the changes were beneficial, and included the addition of knowledge and healing skills the teachers had learned from other systems or had acquired from inner guidance. However, some changes were restrictive, making it more difficult for students to progress.

Some took the Third Degree and divided it into several small parts, calling each new part a new Degree and charging additional money. Often, the fact that they had modified the Usui system was not mentioned and when their students became teachers, they began teaching what they thought was pure Usui Reiki when in fact it was not. In this way, many varieties of Reiki have developed with some thinking they have the only authentic version of Reiki when actually what they are teaching is a modified form. We do not know what happened to the Japanese Techniques?

Mrs. Takata did not teach the techniques with the Japanese names, but she did teach most of them. In the copy of the book entitled "Reiki, a Memorial to Takatai" which included Dr. Hayashi's manual in old Japanese kanji, with a translation. There are notes for first and second degree from one of her students. When comparing the techniques and presentation of material it is virtually the same as Usui and Hayashi Sensei's.

Translation of the Usui Memorial at Saihoji Temple, Tokyo Japan, Rick Rivard provides the following explanation before the translation begins. This is a fairly literal translation of the Usui memorial, as we wanted you, the reader, to get as close a rendition to plain English as possible, without any paraphrasing. This allows you to decide how you would rephrase sentences and paragraphs. There are a few phrases that we haven't translated yet. All comments in (brackets) are either our translations of previous kanji (in quotations), or our explanation of previous words. Please note: there are no periods or paragraphs on the original, so we have added these in to make it easier to read. Also, as in all translations, we had several choices of words for each kanji, and tried to pick what we felt best. Our thanks to Melissa Riggall, Miyuki Arasawa, Yukio Miura and Mr. Hiroshi Doi for their corrections offered.

Translation begins

Memorial of Usui 's "Kudoku"(benevolence)
("kudoku"="koh"+"toku","toku"   that   people experience by culture and training, and "koh" that people practice teaching and the way to save people).

Only the person who has high virtue and does good deeds can be called a great founder and leader. From ancient times, among wise men, philosophers, geniuses and (a phrases that means - very straight and have the right kind of integrity), the founders of a new teaching or new religion are like that. We could say that Usui was one of them.

Usui "Sensei" (literally "he who comes before", thus teacher, or respected person) newly started the method that would change mind and body for better by using universal power. People hearing of his reputation and wanting to learn the method, or who wanted to have the therapy, gathered around from all over. It was truly prosperous.

Sensei's common name is Mikao and other name was Gyoho (perhaps his spiritual name). He was born in the Taniai-mura (village) in the Yamagata district of Gifu prefecture (Taniai is now part of Miyama Village). His ancestor's name is Tsunetane Chiba (a very famous Samurai from the 8th century). His father's name was Uzaemon. His mother's maiden name was Kawai.

Sensei was born in the first year of the Keio period, called Keio Gunnen (1865), on August 15th. From what is known, he was a talented and hard working student. His ability was far superior. After he grew up, he traveled to Europe, America and China to study (yes, it actually says that!). He wanted to be a success in life, but couldn't achieve it; often he was unlucky and in need. But he didn't give up and he disciplined himself to study more and more.

One day he went to Kuramayama to start an asceticism (it says "shyu gyo" - a very strict process of spiritual training using meditation and fasting). On the beginning of the 21st day, suddenly he felt one large Reiki over his head and he comprehended the truth. At that moment he got Reiki "Ryoho" (healing method).

When he first tried this on himself, then tried this on his family, good results manifested instantly. Sensei said that it is much better to share this pleasure with the public at large than to keep this knowledge to our family. So he moved his residence to Harajuku, Aoyama, Tokyo. There he founded "Gakkai" (a learning society) to teach and practice Reiki Ryoho in April of the 11th year of the Taisho period (1921). Many people came from far and wide and asked for the guidance and therapy, and even lined up outside of the building.

September of the twelfth year of the Taisho period (1923), there were many injured and sick people all over Tokyo because of the Kanto earthquake and fire. Sensei felt deep anxiety. Everyday he went around in the city to treat them. We could not count how many people were treated and saved by him. During this emergency situation, his relief activity was that of reaching out his hands of love to suffering people. His relief activity was generally like that.

After that, his learning place became too small. In February of the 14th year of the Taisho period (1925), he built and moved to a new one outside Tokyo in Nakano. (Nakano is now part of Tokyo). Because his fame had risen still more, he was invited to many places in Japan, often. In answering those requests, he went to Kure, then to Hiroshima, to Saga and reached Fukuyama. It was during his stay in Fukuyama that he unexpectedly got sick and died. He was 62 years old. (We think this should be 60 - born August 15, 1865; died March 9, 1926 as per his grave marker).

His wife was from Suzuki family; her name was Sadako. They had a son and a daughter. The son's name was Fuji who carried on the Usui family (meaning the property, business, family name, etc. Born in 1907, at the time of his father's death Fuji was 19. We do know now that Fuji also taught Reiki in Taniai village).

Sensei was very mild, gentle and humble by nature. He was physically big and strong yet he kept smiling all the time. However, when something happened, he prepared towards a solution with firmness and patience. He had many talents. He liked to read, and his knowledge was very deep of history, biographies, medicine, theological books like Buddhism Kyoten (Buddhist bible) and bibles (scriptures), psychology, jinsen no jitsu (god hermit technique), the science of direction, ju jitsu, incantations (the "spiritual way of removing sickness and evil from the body"), the science of divination, physiognomy (face reading) and the I Ching. I think that Sensei's training in these, and the culture which was based on this knowledge and experience, led to the key to perceiving Reiho (short for "Reiki Ryoho"). Everybody would agree with me.

Looking back, the main purpose of Reiho was not only to heal diseases, but also to have right mind and healthy body so that people would enjoy and experience happiness in life. Therefore when it comes to teaching, first let the student understand well the Meiji Emperor's admonitory, then in the morning and in the evening let them chant and have in mind the five precepts which are:

> *First we say, today don't get angry.*
> *Secondly we say, don't worry.*
> *Third we say, be thankful.*
> *Fourth we say, endeavor your work.*
> *Fifth we say, be kind to people.*

This is truly a very important admonitory. This is the same way wise men and saints disciplined themselves since ancient times. Sensei named these the "secret methods of inviting happiness", "the spiritual medicine of many diseases" to clarify his purpose to teach. Moreover, his intention was that a teaching method should be as simple as possible and not difficult to understand. Every morning and every evening sit still in silence with your hands in prayer and chant the precepts, then a pure and healthy mind would be nurtured. It was the true meaning of this to practice this in daily life, using it. (I.e. put it into practical use) This is the reason why Reiho became so popular.

Recently the world condition has been in transition. There is not little change in people's thought. (I.e. it's changing a lot) Fortunately, if Reiho can be spread throughout the world, it must not be a little help (i.e. it's a big help) for people who have a confused mind or who do not have morality. Surely Reiho is not only for healing chronic diseases and bad habits.

The number of the students of Sensei's teaching reaches over 2,000 people already. Among them senior students who adhered in Tokyo are carrying on Sensei's learning place (Dr. Hayashi took title to the school in November, 1926 and together with Mr. Taketomi and Mr. Gyuda, re-located it to Shinano Machi in 1926, and ran it as a hospice) and the others in different provinces also are trying to spread Reiki as much as possible. Although Sensei died, Reiho has to be spread and to be known by many people in the long future. Aha! What a great thing that Sensei has done to have shared this Reiho, which he perceived himself, to the people unsparingly. Now many students converged at this time and decided to build this memorial at Saihoji Temple in the Toyotama district (boundaries have changed and the temple is now in Suginami district) to make clear his benevolence and to spread Reiho to the people in the future. I was asked to write these words. Because I deeply appreciate his work and also I was moved by those thinking to be honored to be a student of Sensei, I accepted this work instead of refusing to do so. I would sincerely hope that people would not forget looking up to Usui with respect .

Composed by "ju-san-i" (subordinate third rank, the Junior Third Court (Rank) -- an honorary title), Doctor of Literature, Masayuki Okada. Written (brush strokes) by Navy Rear Admiral, "ju-san-i kun-san-tou ko-yon-kyu"(subordinate third rank, the Junior Third Court (Rank), 3rd order of merit, 4th class -- again, an honorary title) Juzaburo Gyuda (also pronounced Ushida). Second Year of Showa (1927), February

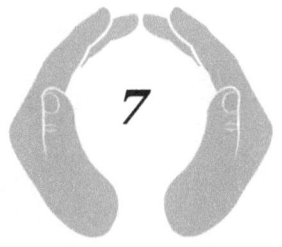

7   *Reiki Energy*

"Reiki" (pronounced "Ray-Key") is a term baptized by Mikao Usui to refer a system of healing which purifies and edifies individuals. When we amalgamate the words "Rei" and "Ki" of Japanese language it becomes "Reiki". In Japanese dictionary 'Rei' mentioned as 'spirit or spiritual' and 'Ki' implies 'energy'. Gist of the word 'Reiki' indicates Universal Life Force Energy. Reiki is the one and only healer, Channel is only an instrument in the healing process.

Reki treatment procedure is very simple. There is no need of removing the clothing of the patient and no undue movement. The person who has empowered vital energy is a Reiki Channel. Reiki is mainly applied via hands. Reiki can be summarized as 'relief from the fingertips'.

He simply places the hands in different spots of the body; subsequently energy emits through the hand and impetuously gives relaxing cum meditating effect to the receiver and giver. The Healer does not need to diagnose diseases but only apprehends balance or imbalance of the body. The energy is therefore given to those lopsided spots by simply placing your hands on yourself for self-treatment (This is also same while treating others).

The Energy thus received sooner or later will balance itself in the body. This is the process of healing via Reiki. There is immortal exhortation about Reiki by Takatai: *"Hands on Reiki on, Hands off, Reiki off"*. Always practice Reiki in a peaceful atmosphere without many disturbances.

Salient Features

1. The character of Reiki energy is divinity and love.
2. Reiki is multifaceted dynamo- as a Self-healing technique and also to heal others.
3. Reiki is a complete therapy and act also as a complementary therapy with other medical systems.
4. Reiki's nature itself is constructive therefore negativity cannot taint it.
5. Reiki can treat patients physically as well as distantly. In distant treatment, patient's physical presence is not needed; it showers to the spot wherever receiver inhabits and usher healing. This is one of the masterstrokes of Reiki.
6. Reiki Attunement remains a lifetime; hence it does not fade away even though you are not utilizing it for several years. We can avail it whenever it is needed.
7. Reiki sheaths the student from pathetic situations because it is at the same time knowledge and also a therapy for healing.
8. Reiki is not only for curing the diseases but also for fulfilling higher objectives in spiritual realms.
9. Reiki can be learned by anybody. It is minus religion, sex or age barriers.
10. Mastering Reiki techniques is lucid and Reiki healing is naive. There is no other system in medical science, which is amusingly simple as Reiki, it can be mastered in a few days' time, and the knowledge about anatomy is least essential, but it will be added advantage, if you have the basic information.
11. Reiki enhances the immunity power and act as a citadel against maladies so it is extremely fruitful to a patient as well as fit person's to sustain optimum health.
12. Reiki can be given to dying patient; even if the receiver does not gain his life, still relives symptoms, shrinks pain, eases emotional distress and in the appropriate time assists the patient in accepting the death peacefully.
13. Reiki can be given to plants and animals, water, rechargeable battery, tea, coffee etc. If Reiki is given to food particles, then it removes all   the   negativity in the food and also en-

hances the taste. Medicines too can be charged with Reiki. (If it is Ayurveda then much better)

Limitations of Reiki

Reiki is always positive; it has no side effects, therefore Reiki is always basking on the safe side. Dr. Subhash Gokhale who is an eye surgeon since '1968; in the past has been assistant professor at Nair Hospital, associate professor at Sion Hospital and head of the department at the Rajeev Gandhi Medical College. He said; "While the medical community is naturally skeptical about this and other forms of alternative healing methods, patients are more open to trying them out. Even if Reiki doesn't work, it can do them no harm. Patients at least are willing to give Reiki a chance". Dr. Subhash Gokhale not only cures patients with Reiki, but spends time convincing a skeptical medical community about its benefits.

Unlike other treatments Reiki has no limitations, but there are some things should be analyzed upon. Some times it heals miraculously and sometimes there is no 'cure'. Thus be ready to cope with any condition.

In cases, which need emergency medical attention such as accidents, bleeding, heart attack etc; it is advisable to consult the medical professional before starting the Reiki treatment. It can act in all these cases, but it is better to give additional treatments along with Reiki.

All diseases cannot be cured in a single session; some- times it may take weeks or even months. Normally, it is necessary to have several treatment sessions for a complete cure; despite the healer's advice, if the patient or his relatives are reluctant to continue more than one treatment or the stipulated sessions, then the diseases are not going to get fully cured. Hence they are more responsible than healer for the end result.

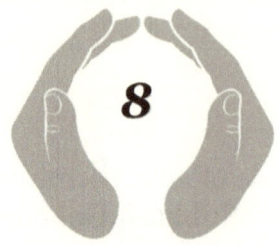

8 Reiki Levels

There are three levels in Reiki. First level is Shoden; Second level is Okuden and Master level is Shinpiden. Master level is sub divided by some masters into two or three levels.

Shoden

In the first level, the healing power will be less when compared to the second level. There is a general saying, you can tap only 20% vital healing energy in the first level and 100% in the second level. This is the seeker level.

Okuden

It is the second level in Reiki levels. There should at least 21 days gap between first and second level. In this level, we are attuned with Three Reiki symbols. It is true that we will become original Reiki channel in this level only. As mentioned earlier it is 20% in the first level and 100% in this level. We obtain most of the sensations at this level. This is the student level.

Shinpiden

There are two symbols in the master level. The gap between second and master level cannot be determined. Only those have five years of healing experience should be given master level. I am in a firm opinion that those who conduct healing in a professional way or those who healing others only is eligible for master level. This level is only for master healers not for normal students.

Grand Master

1. This level is for teaching Reiki. This is again sub divided into three.
2. Study the procedures for healing and first level attunement.
3. Study the procedures for second level attunement.
4. Study the procedures for master level attunement.

Attunement

Reiki cannot be studied from books; it is attained through initiation from Reiki Master. Attunement is the main thing in Reiki. It is a sacred technique that is passed over and over from competent master to the student. If a person is attuned to Reiki, then he/she get connect with the healers leading back to the founder of the system of Reiki. Thus all lineages would lead back to Dr. Usui.

Reiki is above our intellect and logic. It transcends our analysis, so, we cannot be certain about, how and why attunement works. When this energy is properly channelized, it enables us to heal the diseases. By attunement, the student will get the power to channelize the divine energy, or, we are attuned to the healing frequencies. For example, although there are zillion of signals in the atmosphere, we will not get a particular channel by just switching on the TV screen. To obtain it, we have to receive the signals via satellite, and transmit it through excellent cables to the TV screen.

Likewise here in Reiki, healer is receiving the energy by attunement (just like satellite) and transfer it to the patient in the healing session (just like a cable) so his responsibility is limited. He is only a radiant channel and not an ultimate healer. Thus, from this example we can understand that, when these signals are tuned in a particular frequency, then, a particular channel is obtained. There will not be any benefit, if it is not tuned. Hence, we have to tune to that particular frequency for obtaining that particular channel or a radio station. Attunement is also similar to this example. The process by which the student is tuned to that frequency of divine energy is known as attunement.

Attunement generate 21 days of cleansing procedure. There are seven chakras in the body; each chakra needs at least 3 days for cleaning that is how it comes to 21 days. In that period different types of toxins will be released, it may cause loose motions, cold, fever, reddish brown urine, emotional feelings, laughing, crying, anger, greed and lust etc. Thus drink lot of energized water to facilitate the bodies on going toxins rather than trying new medications. This procedure is known as healing crisis.

Benefits of daily treatments

We should practice Reiki in a regular basis. It does not mean to practice daily but it will be fabulous if practiced daily otherwise try to practice at least two times a week or at least one in a week. If you cannot practice it, then there is no need to take Reiki initiation. While giving treatment to other person you will also get healing but the percentage will be less when compared to self treatment.

Do not endure lame excuses for not taking self treatment. We have to create time if it is not getting. Gandhiji said "you will create time to eat your food even in tight schedules and make lame excuses for not getting time to exercise". Time will be there if you have the will do it, so the major obstacle is this laziness. You are not getting the time because you are not fascinated in doing it. Get up little early in the morning than you normal do then you will have enough time to do what ever you like. The major hurdle to get up in the early morning is because the late timing of getting to bed in the night.

In the daily treatment, you will be filled with the Reiki high vibrations and surrounded by it too. This means low vibration energy cannot come close to you, therefore you are protected and this is an important factor.

There are immense benefits from self treatment. Most of them are same characteristics of Reiki treatment mentioned in the topic "Reiki channel". Any way some are mentioned once again.

1. The major one is your energy level will never deplete even though we are meshed in lethargic works.
2. The chance of getting disease now or in future is minimized. All future serious disease will adhere in seed form long before its projection in the body. When they get necessary soil to grow they will grow thickly, and at the appropriate time it will burst out. During that time the root (cause of diseases) will be deep enough to destroy the whole tree (body). Daily treatments enable us to burn the seed from the body because Reiki has the unique quality to treat illnesses and disturbances in the body long before we are aware of any physical problems.
3. Subtle bodies will be strong like a citadel and no disease can penetrate through it.
4. New tissues, cells and hormones will be created and all blockages are removed and create harmony which strengthens the immunity.
5. Mental and emotional worries which are the major cause of serious decease will come under scrutiny.
6. Mind will be calm after the worries disappear which enables to maintain a Robust health.
7. It will give strength to face any events in the life.
8. Improves our concentration.
9. Chances of getting diseases of the patient are inhibited.
10. Amplifies the healing power.

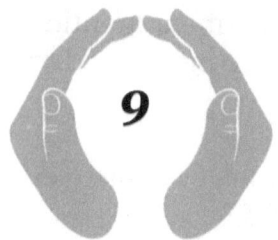

9   *Qualifications*

Even though there is no qualification to Reiki because there is no bar of sex, religion, age, and any educational qualification. But there are some other qualifications, which need to be fulfilled.

Disciples who submit themselves to Reiki should conserve vital energies, speak the truth, refrain from envy and wrath, observe non-violence and should be vegetarian in his life. The methodology of Reiki asserts that the student should act without sycophancy, jealousy, ambition or impudence, never making an exhibition of knowledge and act only with care, affection, and compassion.

His physical outfit should be clean and modest, and speech should be pleasant by using useful and measured words, pure and truthful, never use harsh words or unkind remarks. He should refrain from shabby dealings, committing adultery or covet another's property and should not smoke, take drugs, alcohol or any mind-altering substances. His behavior should never directly or indirectly cause harm to the teacher or others. In addition to these, there are other conditions to pursue, in order to obtain Reiki Empowerment, they are:

1. The student should have the conviction and confidence in Reiki which is the most significant feature. It is not necessary that the patient should require any faith or confidence in Reiki; sometimes the patient may be in ICU or in a COMA state while healing. It can be given to children, plants, animals, etc. Consequently, there is no need to have faith in Reiki during the initial stages of healing. On most occasions it is seen that the person gains confidence and faith in heal-

ing after two or three sessions. Faith is not compulsory for healing but it is essential for obtaining empowerment. The person should possess the confidence and loyalty in Reiki before getting attuned. Hence the best thing is; first heal the student and let him know the sooth- ing effect of Reiki. By obtaining the results, the confidence and loyalty in Reiki will automatically be nurtured. Subsequently, empowerment can be given.(this procedure was followed by Usui and Hayashi Sensei)

2. Students should be free from blocks either mental or physical. If they have blocks, first heal them and then give empowerments.

3. Learning Reiki alone cannot make for an advantage; you have to practice it daily or alternatively. Transform your life with Reiki by avoiding certain things, and prefer positive things (which help to enhance the healing skill). If you have no time or attitude to do all this, do not try to study it. If you have surrendered to it, and have genuine reasons for lack of time for daily practice then it is amend- able. The important thing is the attitude towards Reiki rather than practice.

4. Empowerment should not be given to the students who are reluctant to pay the fees to the Reiki Mas- ter. Even though money is not that relevant, still Reiki Masters are charging the fees in behest to value the levels (which was the principle followed by Mrs.Takata). Empowerments are considered sa- cred, therefore students have an obligation to the Reiki Master; and by paying the fees, and student is evading karmic debts, which otherwise will take births to elude this debt.

5. Empowerment cannot be given to those students whose motive is only to get name, fame or money. His intention to learn Reiki should be unconditional.

6. Anything given freely is always condemned. First of all, Reiki is given as well as taken; we give energy and the patients take energy. The disciple or the healer should think practically while charging the fees. We are not charged for energy because it is free; our charge is for the establishment

cost and the facilities given plus the human effort. Charge the fees according to the patient's financial capacity. If the patient is rich, charge him high and if the patient is poor, charge nominal fees. Money should not be greater criteria to give Reiki or teaching Reiki system, at the same time the receiver should value the healing and training and should not take it as something that is obtained cheaply.

AVOID

After initiation, we should avoid certain things, which will enhance our healing abilities. Bad habits should be avoided otherwise it will be arduous to control. We will lose the moral ability to advice. If we have bad habits, how can we give advice to the patient or student to avoid it? Vegetarianism will healer. Bakery items and fast foods are injurious to health. Eat natural food as possible without color and chemicals. Drink only boiled water. Avoid the following:

1. Bad habits such as Alcohol, Cigarettes, Drugs and using Tobacco products
2. Avoid or Reduce non-vegetarian foods. Strictly avoid red meats such as beef, cow etc.
3. Foods that contain color flavors and Chinese salt
4. Bakery foods which contained fried items
5. Ice-cold foods and drinks.
6. Tinned foods
7. Colas
8. Chocolates
9. Reduce coffee and tea
10. Maida, Rava
11. Refined or hydrogenated oil(use coconut oil)
12. News or Events in TV, Newspaper or in any medium which causes disturbance in your mind.
13. Never eat food or cook food in front of the TV because there will be radiation emitting from it.

All great leaders said us to avoid these things. Swami Vivekananda said; "All fried items are really poisonous. The sweets from the vendor's shop are death's door. The spices are no food at all; to take them in abundance is only due to bad habit". "Fermented bread is poison. Do not touch it all. Flour mixed with yeast becomes injurious. Never take fermented thing. In this respect the prohibition in our Shastras of partaking of any such article of food are of great importance. Any sweet thing, which has turned sour, is called by Shastras as "shukta" and that is prohibited to take, expect buttermilk, which is good and beneficial. If you have to take bread, toast it well over the fire". He also said," Too much of oily and fatty food produces fat in the body.

Mahatma Gandhi said; "All condiments, even salt, destroy the natural flavor of the foodstuff much more than after the addition of salt or other condiments. Several condiments are not required by the body as a general rule, e.g., chillies fresh or dry, pepper, turmeric, coriander, caraway, mustard, methi, asafoetida, etc. These are taken just for the satisfaction of the palate.

"People use tobacco for smoking, snuffing and also for chewing. As for chewing tobacco, it is the dirtiest of all the three ways in which tobacco is used. Lovers of health, if they are slaves to any of these evil habits, will resolutely get out of the slavery. All the three are the dirtiest habits".

"Tea, Coffee and Cocoa are not required by the body. Hot water, honey and lemon make a healthy nourishing drink, which is a well substitute for tea or coffee".

"Smoking causes salivation and most smokers have no hesitation in spitting anywhere. There is no doubt that tobacco is an intoxicant and while under its effects one forgets one's worries and misfortunes".

"Alcohol makes a man forget himself and while its effects last, he becomes utterly incapable of doing anything useful. Those who take to drinking ruin themselves and ruin their people. They lose all sense of decency and propriety".

In a nut shell, alcohol creates a physical, moral, economical & intellectual imbalance in a person. Tobacco has sim- ply worked havoc among mankind. Once caught in its tangle, it is rare to find anyone to get out of it again. Tolstoy has called it the worst of all intoxicants. Tobacco smokers become callous and careless of others' feeling.

Proper diet

"Eat to live, not live to eat", is a great proverb to remember because it is the food which makes us the diseases as well as robust health. A good diet enhances health, whereas a bad diet results in diseases. Subsequently, health depends upon what you eat. Ayurveda says, the order in which we eat different classes of foods, how we combine them, and the amount

We consume determines how well we digest and assimilate our vital nutrients. The better we digest and assimilate our foods, the less likely are we to form toxic substances, accumulate excess fat, and crave unhealthy food articles. Ayurveda offers a rational and scientific approach for determining correct diet, which is based upon an individual's constitution.

According to Ayurveda, every food has its own taste (Rasa), a hot or cold energy (Veerya) and post-digestive effect (Vipaka). When two or three different food substances are of different taste, the energy and the post-digestive effect com- bines together & Agni becomes overloaded, inhibiting the en- zyme system and resulting in production of toxins in the sys- tem. Thus, according to Ayurveda, one should eat according to one's constitution and take fruits, starches, proteins and fats separately at different times of the day. It is the quality that is important than quantity. Hence we cannot say that a person who ate a full stomach is in good health.

Food should be simple and naturally delicious. When the diet is eaten in an enjoyable atmosphere, and as an offer- ing; which also have a proper mixture of fibers, fats, proteins, vitamins, carbohydrates and minerals, that food alone can be termed as quality food. So try to include as many vegetables especially leafy vegetables, fruits and grains in the diet. These foods are enriched with fibers, which helps in the elimination of waste products from the body. The consumption of it provides additional amount of fats, proteins, carbohydrates, vitamins and minerals needed by the body. Orange, Banana, Chickoo, Green leafy vegetables like spinach; Cabbage, etc., are a very rich source of essential vitamins and minerals to the body.

In olden days man used to prepare natural and unprocessed foods and they made it in a simple way. By assimilating these simple foods, our physiology functioned at a paramount. The basic difference between our times and olden times are that, they only ate two or three different types of foods at a time. We tend to have maximum types or at least six or seven types of food at most meals. When we consume numerous types of food at a single meal, then, it will be very arduous for our digestive glands to manufacture, and secrete many different digestive enzymes simultaneously. This westernization of foods have spoiled us and made us ill. Swami Vivekananda said, "Imitate their (traditional) food as much as you can, the more you lean westwards to copy the modes of food, the worse you are, and the more uncivilized you become".

We also eat many times today than in olden days. We eat food all the time, and there are only limited intervals between them. Saints believed to eat only once a day. But it is not possible for the ordinary man. So, how often should one eat? Gandhiji said, "Many people take two meals a day. The general rule is to take three meals: breakfast early in the morning and before going out to work, dinner at midday and supper in the evening or late. There is no necessity to have more than three meals". In cities some people keep on nibbling from time to time. This habit is harmful. The digestive apparatus requires rest.

Food should be eaten fresh and as raw as possible. Over cooking and processing can deplete the nutrition in it. If possible, eat in silence. A balanced vegetarian diet provides sufficient quantities of these essential ingredients which are vital for a good health and mental balance. It enables to strengthen the immunity system of body, and thereby reduces the chances of getting ailments. These are absent (particularly fiber which is the essential part of the food) in non-vegetarian food. If you cannot get all those vegetables and fruits, then try to take any one of the following Ayurvedic Rasayanams in a teaspoon. Take only one Rasayana at a particular period of time.

Different qualities in food

1. Fibers are the most important among the foods. The consumption of fiber results in the formation of softer stools; as it absorbs water from the stomach. It helps in the elimination of toxins. It also provides a satiety value to the diet. Fiber content foods are fruits, vegetables and cereals. Ex-oats, carrots, beetroot, pinto beans, brown rice, bananas, wheat breads and in all leafy vegetables. Cereals content foods are:-Rice, Wheat, Bajra, Maize, Jowar, Wheat flour, Rice flakes, etc.

2. Proteins are essential for the maintenance of the tissues.

3. They are also required for the formation of enzymes and hormones. Break down of protein creates nitrogenous waste which effects major organs particularly kidneys. Protein content foods are: soybeans, French beans, milk, seeds, nuts like cashew nut, peanuts, badam etc.

4. Fats provides the body with a reserve of energy, build and maintain cushions for internal organs, make the protective myelin sheaths that encloses the nerve and also supplies a small quantity of vitamins such as A, D, E and K. Fat content foods are: ghee, soybeans, dry coconut, cashew nut, peanuts, and oils.

5. Carbohydrates are the chemical formed in which plants store energy and are recommended as the main source of energy in the diet. They provide energy and should be added bulk in the diet. They also provide roughage, which

is necessary for the elimination of waste. It is also hard to di- gest so always check the digestive capacity and choose the diet accordingly. Carbohydrate content foods are: white rice, wheat, pulses and beans, corn, breads, potatoes, tapiocas and all products grown under the soil.

6. Vitamins and minerals are involved in the utilization of major nutrients like carbohydrates, protein and fats. They are also required to carry out many vital functions in the body. Balance of it regulates the proper functioning of the body. The minerals form the body part's structural component. They act as catalyst's agent in many body reactions. Plants produce vitamins and also take in minerals.

Vitamins and Minerals content foods are:

1. Vitamin-A: Carrot, beetroot, tomato, cauliflower, mango, orange, pineapple, spinach, and different types of leaves.
2. Vitamin-B: peanuts, sprouting seeds, yeast, tomato, orange, cucumber, melons, milk, egg, and vegetables.
3. Vitamin-C: cabbage, cauliflower, amla, lime, drumstick, leaves of radish, tomatoes, Lemons, guava, apples, papaya.
4. Vitamin-D: milk, butter, egg.
5. Vitamin-E: Red pepper, vegetable oils, leaves, wheat leaves.

10   *Daily Routine*

Health is Wealth

Water

Drink at least 10-12 glass water daily, it can be in the form of juices, soups, tea, coffee etc. Do not drink water while you are eating. Drink before or after 30 minutes during the meal. Drinking juices or soups during meal time is good. If possible, try to drink water from the wells or boiled water which is lukewarm. Swami Vivekananda said, "Impure water and impure food are the cause of all maladies"

Food

Swami Vivekananda said "That much one can assimilate is proper food for one. Growing thin or fat is equally due to indigestion". If possible, eat solid food twice a day, and drink juice or soups as the third one. Generally speaking, eating less is good for health. Swami Vivekananda said, "The food should be such that it contains the greatest nutrient in the smallest compass, and at the same time quickly assimilated; otherwise, if taken in larger quantity continuously, the whole day is required only to digest it. If all the energy is spent only on digestion, what will there be left to do the other work".

The ideal combination is; fill half your stomach with solid foods, one-third water, and one-third empty. There should be 4 hours interval between each food, and do not eat in between them, even though it may be light food. Don't fast more than 6 hours. If possible, do not eat solid foods after 8Pm and before 7Am. Avoid eating foods 45 minutes before sunrise and sunset. Don't eat food in the mid noon.

While eating, your mind should be relaxed and food eaten should be as an offering to the body, and for the whole universe. Do not eat in front of TV or Computers. Eating food is considered as an offering to the vital energy, so we should follow these conditions. The food should be cooked and served happily, and the mind should be free off tensions and anxiety.

Tension creates chemicals in the body and the food cooked in a melancholic mood, affects the mind, hence it should be avoided. Never eat in a standing position even though it is a snack, always sit while eating. Do not waste food. Give importance to quality & not quantity. So try to eat vegetables and fruits more. Give a little Reiki in the stomach after your Meals, which will speed up the digestive process.

Sleep

Swami Vivekananda said, "Proper food, proper exercise, proper sleep, and proper wakefulness are necessary for any success" 6 hours sleep daily is a must. One should not adhere to sleepless nights. Avoid sleep during daytime. Do not watch TV or Computer after 10 Pm; and also do not read during these hours. Try to wake up at 5 Am and Sleep at 10 Pm.

Mood

Always be in a relaxed mood. Avoid anger, fear, anxiety, tensions, greed, lust and all those type of emotional and mental feelings. One should be contented with whatever chance may bring to him and adhere to be desire-less. Swami Vivekananda said, "That man alone who is the lord of his mind can become happy and none else".

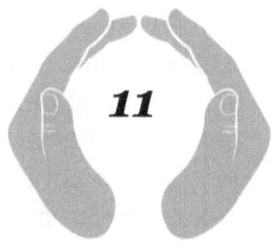

11 *Principles & Prayers*

Reiki principles originally came from Precepts used in 9th century Japanese Buddhism; Usui changed them Regarding dates for when he introduced the present precepts into Reiki teachings, it is known that he was teaching them from early 1915, living proof of this exists. The precepts at that time did not include the first two lines and last two lines. Usui did not devise his Precepts as something to simply believe in but as something to practice in daily life. Every morning and evening, join your hands in prayer. Pray these words to your heart and chant these words with your mouth.

The secret of inviting happiness through many blessings
The spiritual medicine for all illness
For today only: Do not get angry Do not worry
Be humble
Be honest in your work
Be compassionate to yourself and others Do Gassho every morning and evening Keep in your mind and recite.

From Usui's memorial, 'when it comes to teaching, first let the student understand well the Meiji Emperor's admonitory, then in the morning and in the evening let them chant and have in mind the five admonitions which are:

Don't get angry today.
Don't be grievous.
Express your thanks.
Be diligent in your business.
Be kind to others.

The Ideals as taught by Mrs. Takata

> *Just for today, thou shall not anger*
> *Just for today, thou shall not worry*
> *Thou shall be grateful for the many blessings*
> *Earn thy livelihood with honest labor*
> *Be kind to thy neighbors*

Reiki Prayer

> *I Thank Reiki For Being Here*
> *I Thank Dr Usui For Being Here*
> *I Thanks All The Reiki Masters*
> *I Thank Myself*
> *I Thank The Patient*
> *I Thank Reiki*
> *I Thank Reiki*
> *I Thank Reiki*

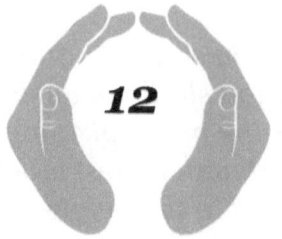

12   *The Procedure*

Healing is more practical than knowledge so we can say that it is a synthesis of esoteric knowledge, which is realized and made practical in a session. It is practice first and knowledge afterward. Reiki is, after all, on the practical side. It deals with healing alone, and theory is only a basic form, so we must make the sharpest distinction between talk and intuitive experience.

If we give thousands of theories about Reiki it will not be sufficient to heal the illness of a patient. It is the Reiki session that cures the diseases and not theories. Therefore, it is neither talk nor theories, nor doctrine; however, great they may be helpful in the practical side of healing. While healing every part of the healer's soul becomes transcended into what it (energy) believes. Therefore, the real work is in the practice. Absorption of ourselves with the healing power is the process happening in a Reiki session.

Always abide these laws in a session. You should give Reiki to a person who has asked for it, and don't refuse it as an inconvenience unless there is a genuine inconvenience from your side. Similarly, never give Reiki to a person who has not requested it. Treat all patients sincerely. If you are sincere, then Reiki energy, which is divine love energy, will flow in a greater alacrity and will enable the patient to recover rapidly. If you are not sincere then the energy flow will be interrupted. Sincerity means you treat the patient with the same spirit as you treat yourself. I think this is the fundamental principle. Always abide and be thankful to Reiki energy that is the real healer and acing. Reiki sessions should be conducted in peaceful surroundings.

Before starting a session, the mood and necessary time for practicing Reiki are important. If the healer is not in the mood then try to avoid the session. The methodology of Reiki session is as follows. First smudge the patient's aura. You can sweep the negative energy of the patient with salt water in a chronic disease. After that sit in a relaxed mood and chant the five principles and prayer of Reiki, then draw the symbols and whisper its sacred name. After that, play slow music or devotional songs for the receiver to obtain a pleasant mood for healing.

Start the treatment by placing the hands on the first position and practice the subsequent positions. For each position, there should be at least three minutes duration. The duration will be increased as per the sensations obtained from that spots. As said before, one has to give energy on those spots till the receiver receives it. When the receiver stops receiving then place your hands on the next position and give energy till he receives and then to the next spot & so on, till the whole body is filled with positive energy.

Chant the prayer after the session. Striking and sealing is not necessary for self-treatment, it is only used when you are treating others. So do them while you practice healing with others. Wash your hands before and after Reiki sessions.

Do the following:

1. Reiki prayer before and after the sessions.
2. Connect to Reiki energy
3. Stroke and seal the patient after the treatment.

Practice Reiki for 21 days & after 21 days you can reduce the hand positions and give only to those portions where energy is needed. Try to practice Reiki in all of your actions, such as eating, drinking, sleeping, discussing, etc. Always remember this quote of Mrs. Takatai *"5 minutes Reiki is better than no Reiki at all"*.

Avoid

1. Reiki should not be taken lightly.
2. Reiki symbols should be kept as sacred and secret. Never disclose them to anyone.
3. Reiki should not be given to a patient unless he asks you to do so, even to the dearest friend nor relatives of the practitioner. Infants and animals have their way of showing disinclination, and if you see such disinclination you should respect and refrain from it.
4. If the patient is angry or violent, under the influence of alcohol, drugs or any other intoxicant, then, treat them only with the consent of relatives, or from the behest of the relatives.
5. If the patient is seriously ill, and should be immediately moved to hospital; in that case, if the relatives make a strong request, and if you have the mental strength and confidence to heal, then proceed; otherwise don't.
6. Never give Reiki reluctantly. If you do not have the mood, or from an intuition not to heal; do not proceed further. In some cases; mainly in chronic diseases, or dying patients they will show some sort of disinclination; either by removing the hand or by verbal deeds, then do not proceed further.
7. Never give Reiki if the patient is showing disrespect.
8. Never give Reiki if the patient is not following your advice
9. Never give Reiki if the patient is reluctant or absent to reach the clinic in time on all days.

13   *Visualizations*

Energy Ball Exercises

Hold your hands so that your palms are facing each other, about two inches apart. Take a few deep breaths, focusing your heed on the space between your hands. Move your palms apart until there is about six inches between them, and then move them forward till they are almost touching. Continue moving them gently, apart and together, for a minute or two. Pay heed to the sensations between your hands. (If after a few minutes of this, you don't feel any sensations, try rubbing your hands together vigorously for a minute, and then repeating this experiment.)

You may feel some tingling or warmth. You may find that at some point, it feels as if there is resistance; it may feel like "the air is thicker" or like there's outward pressure like magnets pushing each other away. This is because you have met the edge of the energy field emanating from the other palm. Gently move the hands a little closer together (about an inch). You may now feel tingling on the back of your hands.

The energy field of each hand has passed through the other hand. Again move them toward each other, until you feel resistance. Imagine this energy is a ball, and curl your fingers around the edges of it. Play with this, moving one palm up along the top side of the ball, while the other moves below, and so on, exploring how the energy feels.

Gassho meditation

Sit calmly with head upright, fold your hands in the Namaste position, concentrate on the middle finger, imagine that there is a balloon in your stomach and inhale deeply to fill the balloon and exhale slowly for a few seconds. Chant the five principles of Reiki and the prayer. Imagine that there is a golden globe above your head. And it is slowly entering into the Crown chakra and from there to Brow chakra, Throat chakra and to Heart chakra.

Then the globe replicates itself into two globs, from there one glob passes through the right lung then the right shoulder, right biceps, right forearm then to the center of the right palm. Similarly the other globe moves from left lung then the left shoulder, left biceps, left forearm then to the center of the left palm. From there the self effulgent and vibrant golden globes merge into one at the center of your palms. It explodes itself into golden vibrating rays and flows through the tips of fingers.

Silva mind meditation

Sit in a comfortable posture. Breathe deeply three times. Concentrate on stomach. Fill it with air and contract it. Do it three to five times. Think we are gone back to heart. After this, imagine that your mind is going up, and leaving the body consciousness. Imagine that, your mind is seeing a vast meadow and a huge tree touching the skies amid of the plane.

Now go near the tree, and request it to allow you to enter its trunk. Then fill in with the vast energy inside the tree into your self. After that, imagine the tree is growing very fast and fills the whole world with its branches and leaves and the roots growing down to the center of the earth. The tree is drawing vast energy and you also start to draw energy accordingly. Now you are filled with full of energy and you are in high spirits. When satisfied, slowly come out of the tree.

Feel grateful to the tree for its generous attitude towards you. Then return to your heart. Feel that you are immersed in energy with peace and happiness.

Other Techniques

There are lots of ancient practices in Tibetan and Yogic system that is taught in my Reiki First Level class for enhancing the Reiki Power. Those techniques are not mentioned in the manual because it should be taught and monitored by a competent master. Get in touch with me to know more about it.

14 ***Hand Positions***

The Reiki Treatments of the First Degree

- Auto-treatment
- Quick treatment
- Chakras balancing treatments
- Treatments of the five organs
- Basic treatment
- Treatments to plants, animal, food and medicines

Everyone can do this treatment to himself. Starting from the head, the hands placed over the various Chakras for o few minutes, as follows:

- Top of the head (VII Chakra)
- Fore Head (VI Chakra)
- Throat (V Chakra)
- Brest (IV Chakra)
- Stomach (III Chakra)
- Belly (II Chakra)
- Pelvis (I Chakra)

Reiki Practice

Reiki energy flows more smoothly and effectively within the patient's body through the practitioner hand, hence a definite sequence hand positions are important. The basic set of hand positions are nearly eighteen for self treatment and nearly twenty two for healing others. These hand positions cover all the major energy channels, chakras and aura.

Hand positions

Before administering any of these positions; hold both hands with palms down, facing the body of the patient. Extend and hold the fingers and thumb together, making an arch, so that a hollow is created under the palms. Splayed fingers or flat palms might allow the energy to dissipate. Do not let the recipient cross his/her legs or arms. Reiki touch is very light, so, no pressure is applied. The energies often run for about 3 to 5 minutes in each position.

Head positions

The head positions; it is considered as the most important positions of the human body. You can evaluate the whole body, and character of the patient from the sensations of the head. You should give treatment to the four head positions to each and every type of diseases regardless whether disease is for head or not. It can be given either by, sitting or standing behind the patient's head. The patient can sit upright on a chair, or lie down on his or her back on a massage table or a mattress placed on the floor. The best way always is in lying down on the massage table.

Position 1: Eye

To treat yourself: Cup the eyes with your palms, with your fingers on the forehead and the sides of your palm comfortably placed on the sides of the nose. Let the smallest finger of each hand meet the third eye.

To treat others: Sit or stand behind the head and place your arched palms on the eyes. The thumbs of both hands should touch near the middle of the eyebrows. Place your fingers comfortably on the sides of the patient's nose, taking care not to hinder or constrict the nostrils.

Position 2: Temples

To treat yourself: Place your palms on your temples (between your eyes and ears). Each palm should be somewhere between the eye and the earlobe.
To treat others: Place your palms on the temples, with the tips of your fingers reaching the cheek bones. Keep your fingers and the thumbs together.

Position 3: Ears

To treat yourself: Place your cupped palms on your ears.
To treat others: Same as above.

Position 4: Occipital Lobes

The occipital lobe is the rearmost lobe in each hemisphere of the brain.

To treat yourself: Cup the occipital lobes where the throat meets the lower back of the skull.
To treat others: Cradle the back of the head in your relaxed palms. The sides of the palms should touch, with the fingers reaching the base of the skull.

Position 5: Throat

To treat yourself: Slide one hand under the hollow of the neck and bring the other over the throat. Keep the fingers and thumbs of both hands together.
To treat others: Same as above. Let the edge of the upper palm take support from the patient's collar bone so he or she does not feel pressure on the wind pipe. Alternately, the palms can be kept at sides of the throat.

Position 6: Shoulders/ Lungs

To treat yourself: place your palms over your shoulders, at the sides of your neck. If you find this difficult, you may cross your arms so that each palm touches the opposite shoulder. Alternately, hold one palm over the opposite shoulder, near the neck, and place the other palm over the kidney on that side. Repeat on the other shoulder. If you adopt this variation, you may skip the kidney position.

To treat others: Place your palms over the shoulders, parallel to each other. Alternately, place your palms in a straight horizontal line across the shoulder blades, with the Fingertips of the hand closer to you touching the heel of the other palm.

Body Positions

Position 7: Heart

To treat yourself: keep your lower hand where it is but move the upper one below it, still adjacent.

To treat others: Same as above. However, when treating a woman, place one hand between the breasts and the other horizontally just above it (over the thymus gland), forming a T. If you are a male and not on intimate terms with your patient, keep your hands an inch or so above the breasts as a mark of respect for woman's privacy. You can also use this T variation for males if your intuition guides you to do so, or if you simply find yourself more comfortable with it. Alternately, place your left palm over your right palm above the heart. Though it is the heart chakra (placed right in the center) and not the physical heart (which is slightly towards one's left), allow your hands to be guided a bit to one side by any pull or repulsion they experience.

Position 8: Solar plexus

To treat yourself: keep your hands above both sides of the navel.
To treat others: Same as above. Alternately, place the hands in a horizontal line across the solar plexus.

Position 9: Liver/Gall bladder/ Pancreas/Spleen

To treat yourself: Keep your hands on both sides of the navel.
To treat others: Same as above. Alternately, place the hands in a horizontal line across the spleen, across the depression where the lower ribs meet in front.

Position 10: Navel/Hara

To treat yourself: Place one hand above the navel and the other below it.
To treat others: Same as above.

Position 11: Groin

To treat yourself: Form a V with your palms over the pelvic bones, and adjust until your hands cover the genitals. Keep your fingers and thumbs together.
To treat others: Same as above, but it might be more convenient to point the forehand in the opposite direction (i.e., point the closer hand towards the things and the farther hand away from them). Preserve your patient's privacy by keeping your hand just above his or her body.

Position 12: Kidneys/adrenal glands

To treat yourself: Place your palms in a horizontal line across your back, one palm width above the waist (in line with the lower ribs), fingertips touching.

To treat others: Same as above, but you may find it more convenient to point the fingertips of the far hand away from you (touch the fingertips of one hand to the heel of the other palm).

Leg positions

You can either treat two knees jointly or separately. If you are doing it separately then hold one hand above the knee and other hand under the knee.

Position 13: Knees

To treat yourself: Assume a sitting posture and cup your knees with your hands.
To treat others: Same as above. Alternately, treat each knee separately by placing both hands on one knee at a time—one above and the other at the back, in the hollow of the Joint. This variation is preferable for those with stiff or weak knee joints, those under stress, those confronting and fearing a particular change in life or those who generally
Find it emotionally difficult to face life's challenges with mettle.

Position 14: Left Foot

To treat yourself: Hold your left foot with both hands in a way that is comfortable.
To treat others: hold the left foot with both hands in a way that is comfortable to you.

Position 15: Left Toes

You can either treat both toes separately or jointly. If you are doing it joints then place your hands on both toes.

To treat yourself: Hold your left toe with both hands in a way that is comfortable.

To treat others: Hold your left toe with both hands in a way that is comfortable.

Positions 16-17: Right Foot and Toes

Repeat positions 16-18 on the left foot. There is no major difference between left and right food in healing.

Back positions

The back represents support, both financial (lower back) and emotional (upper back). Optional one, it is mainly used to treat others; if the client has back problems, asthma, and lung problems. If your intuition indicates to treat back then heal it. The back often receives Reiki when treating front parts of the body.

Position 18: Lungs

It is an optional position for throat. You can skip this if you had treated in the front position of neck (Position: 5)

To treat others: Place your hands on the lungs with palm flat on both sides of the patient.

Position 19: Back of Hara

To treat others: back side of the position 8. Hands can be placed either vertical or horizontal as per your convenience. .

Position 20: Muladharam

To treat others: Place one hand over and along the fold of the buttocks and the other perpendicular to it, forming a T. Be careful while you touch any private parts of others.

Hand Positions

I am deeply thankful to Miss. Santhakumari E N, for sketching Reiki Hand Positions

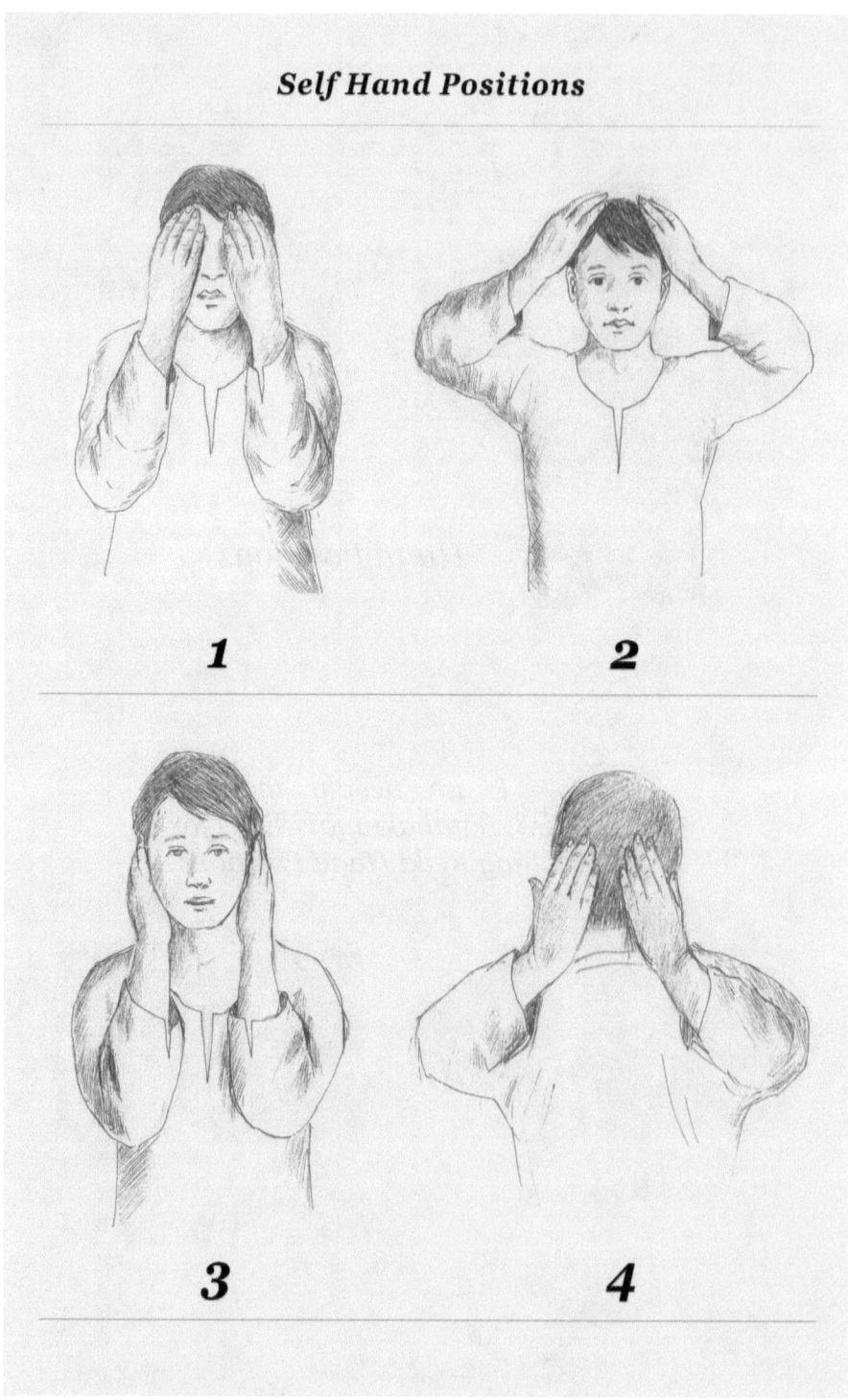

Self Hand Positions

Self Hand Positions

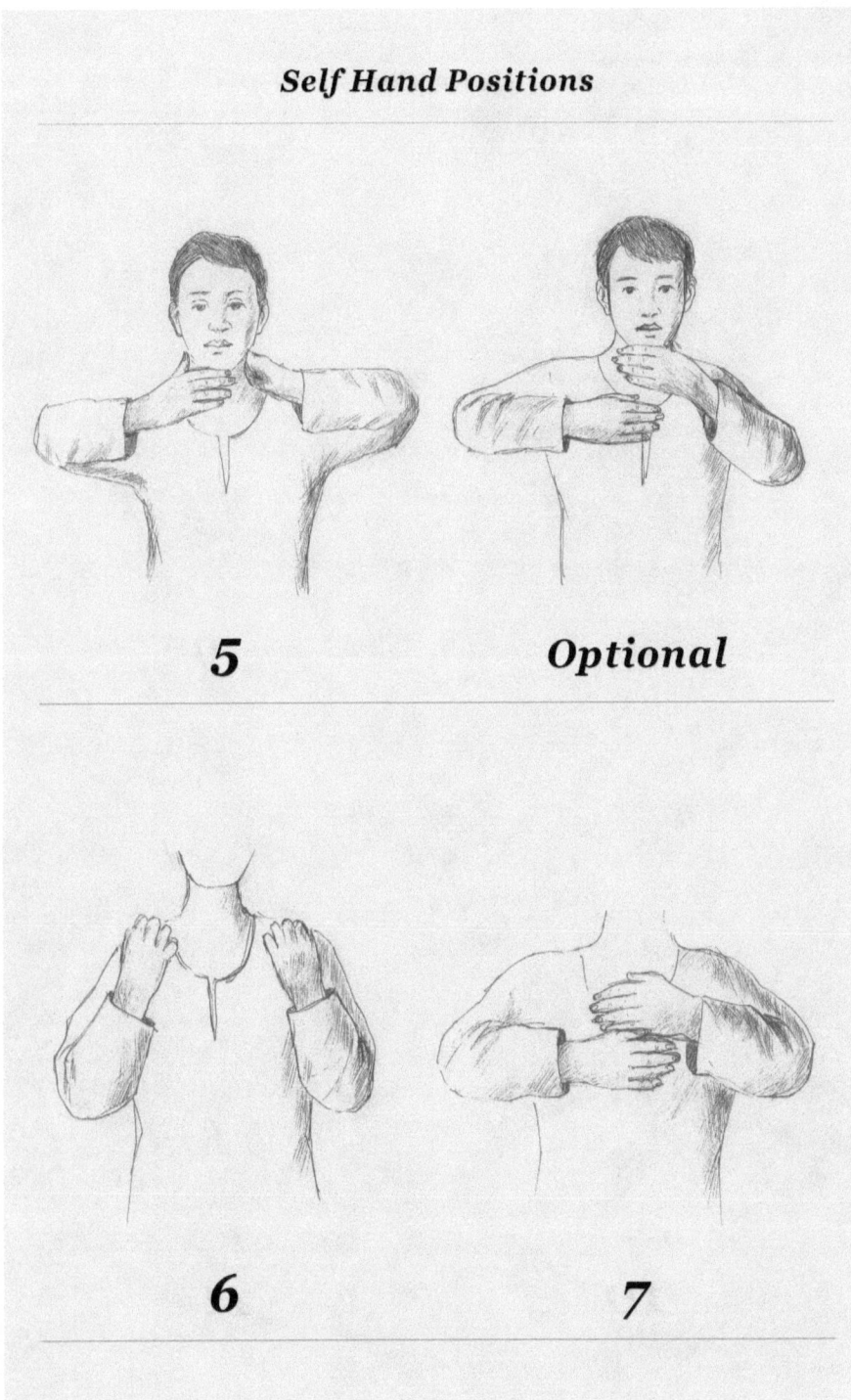

5

Optional

6

7

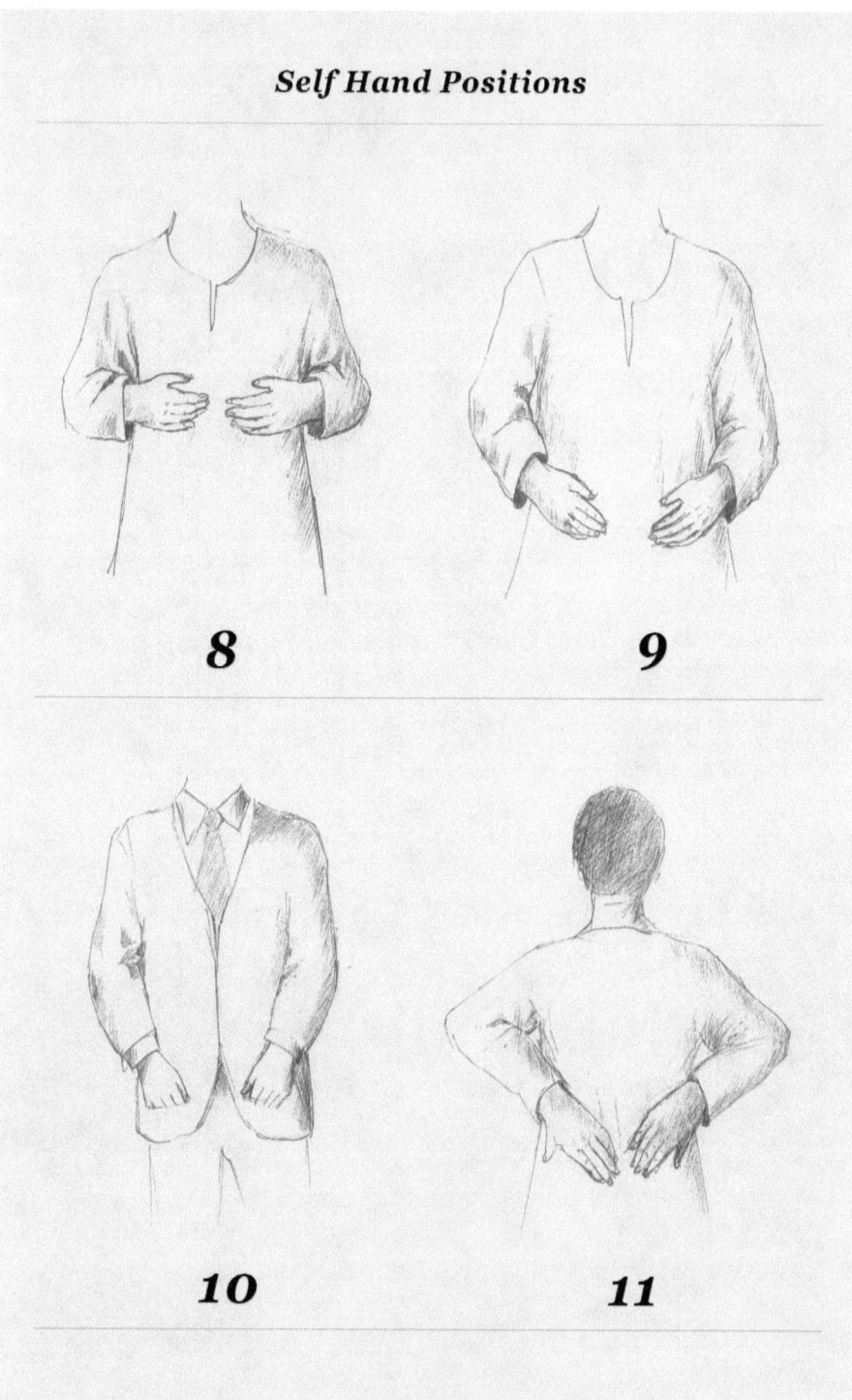

Self Hand Positions

8

9

10

11

Self Hand Positions

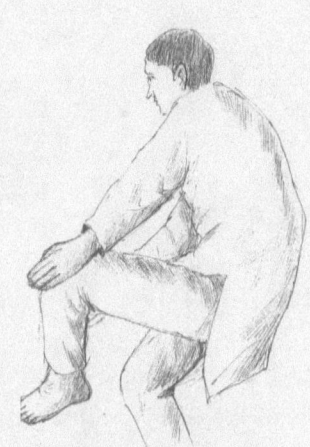

12 & 13

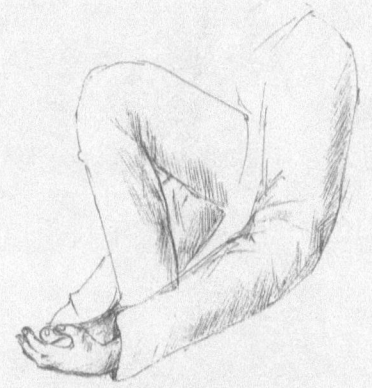

14 & 15

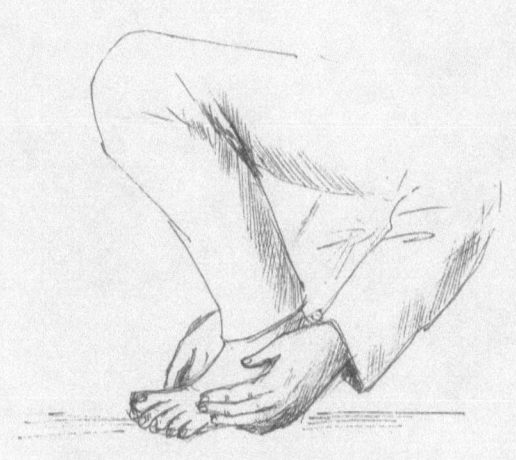

16 & 17

Others - Hand Positions

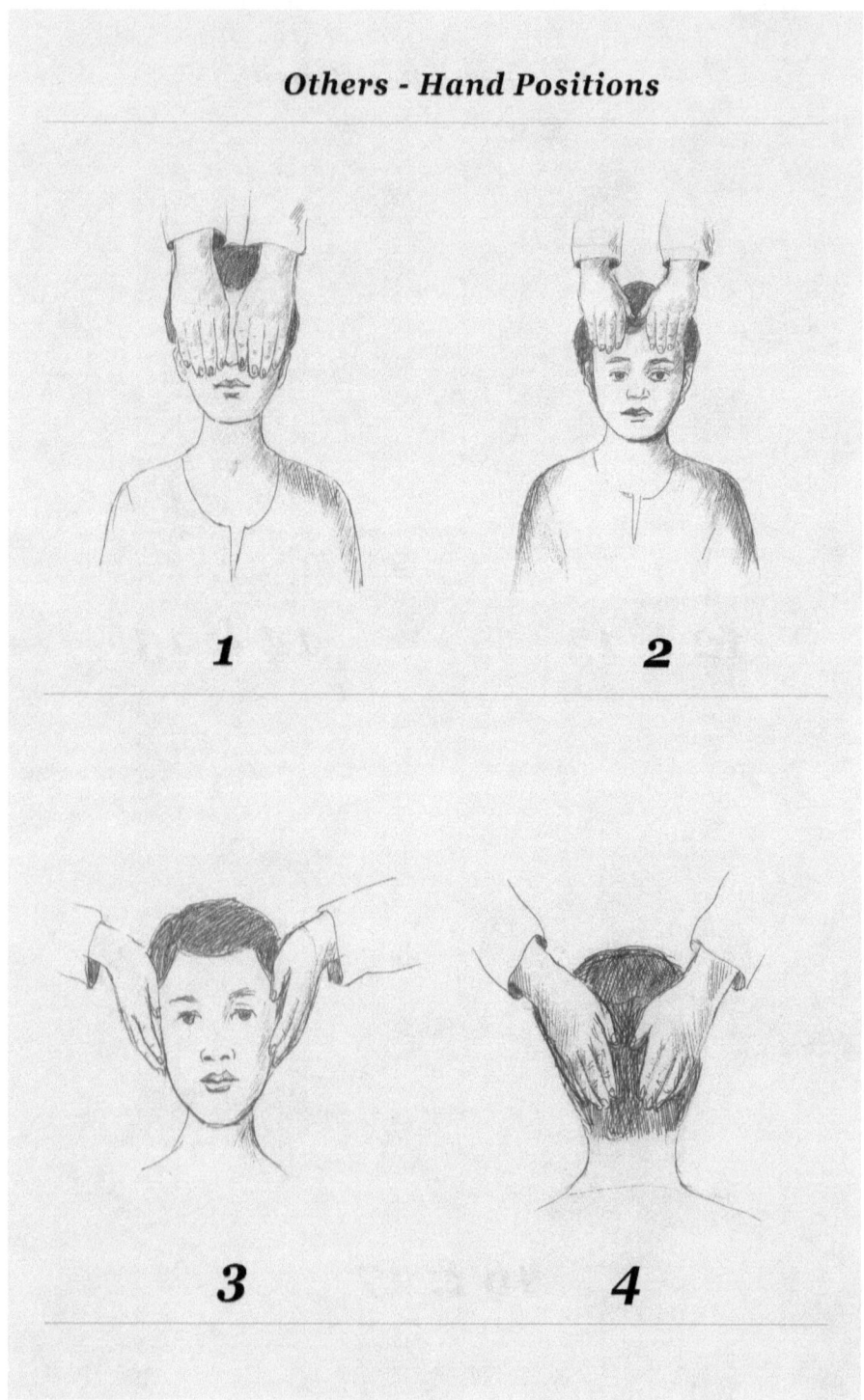

Others - Hand Positions

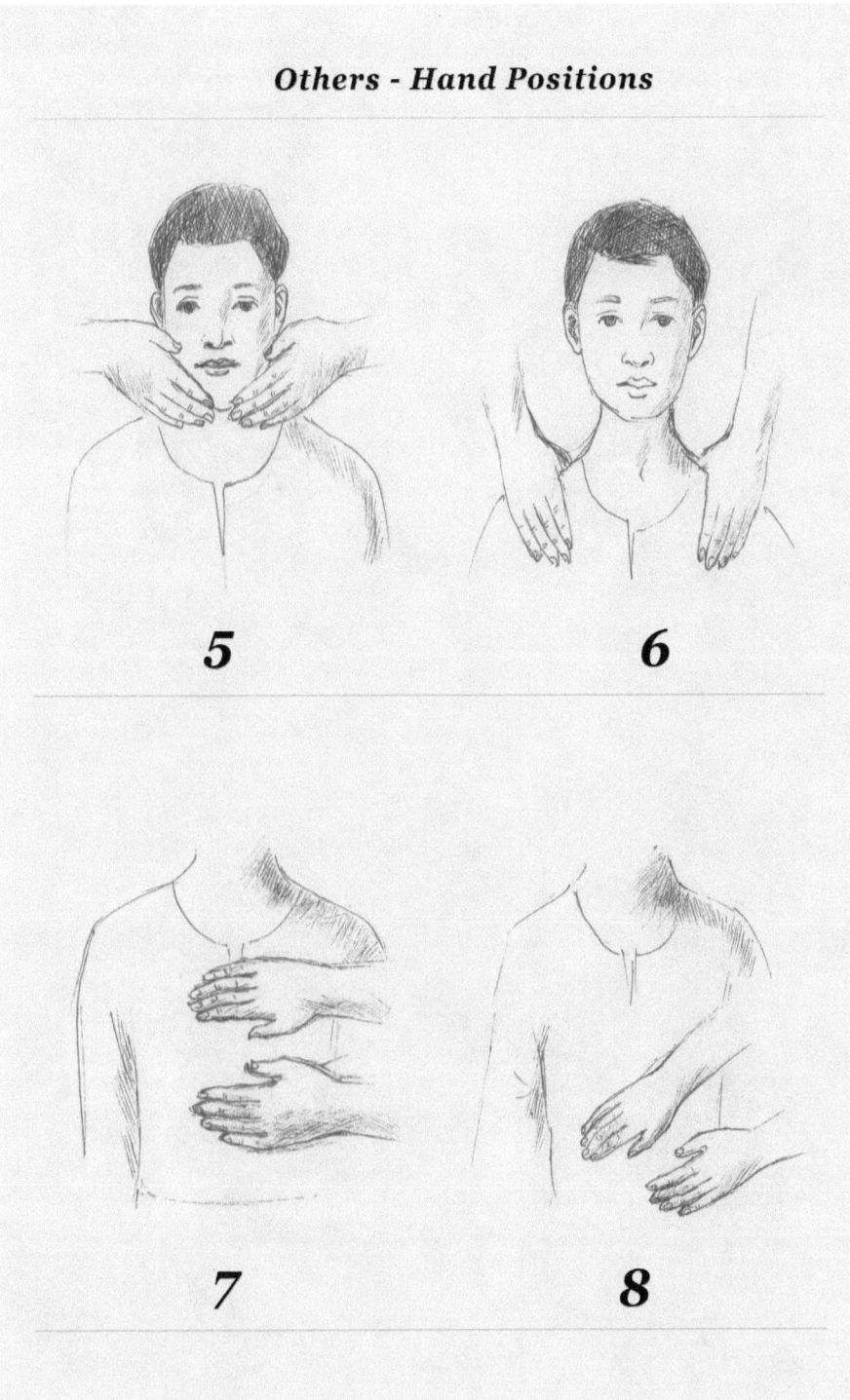

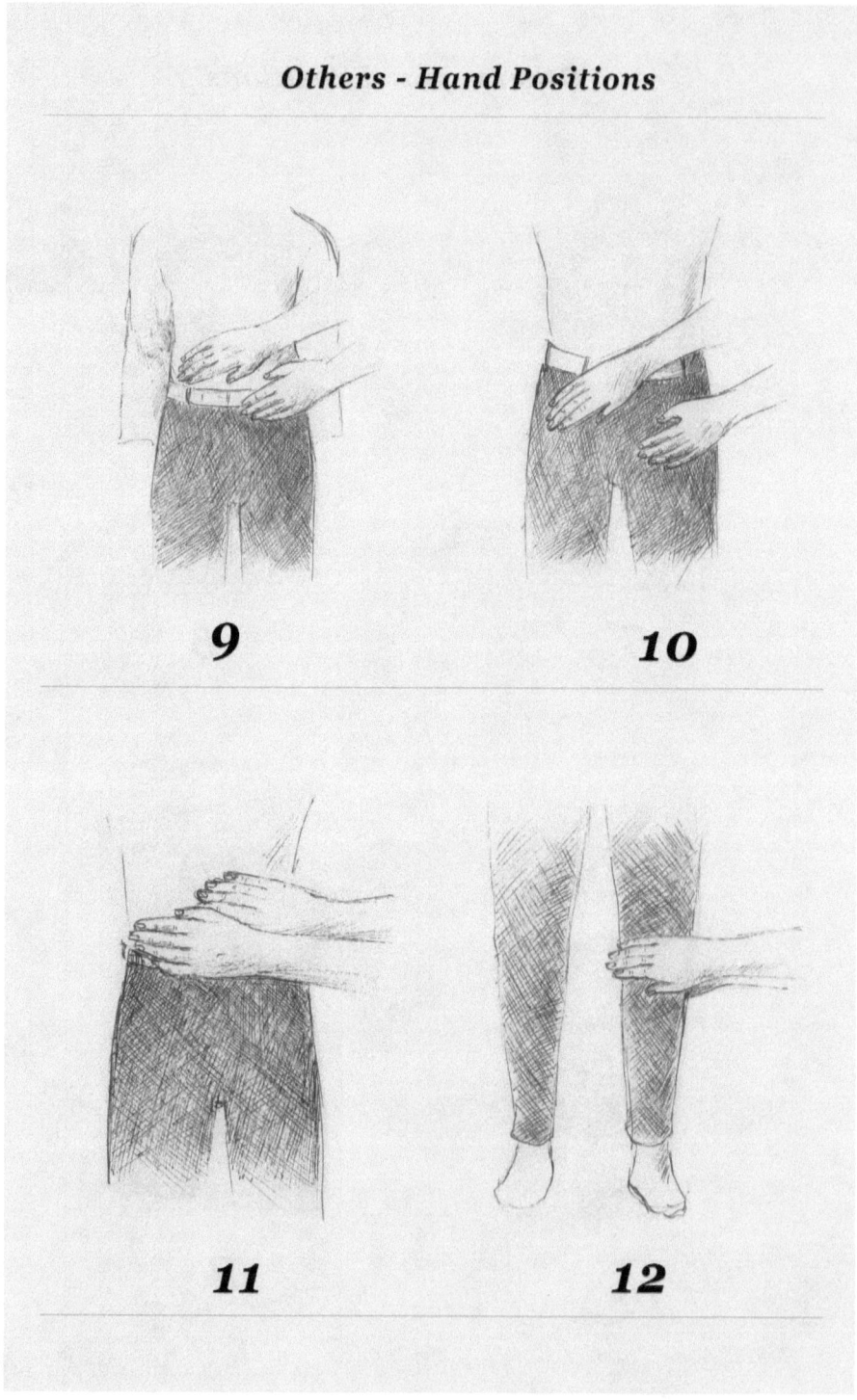

Others - Hand Positions

9

10

11

12

Others - Hand Positions

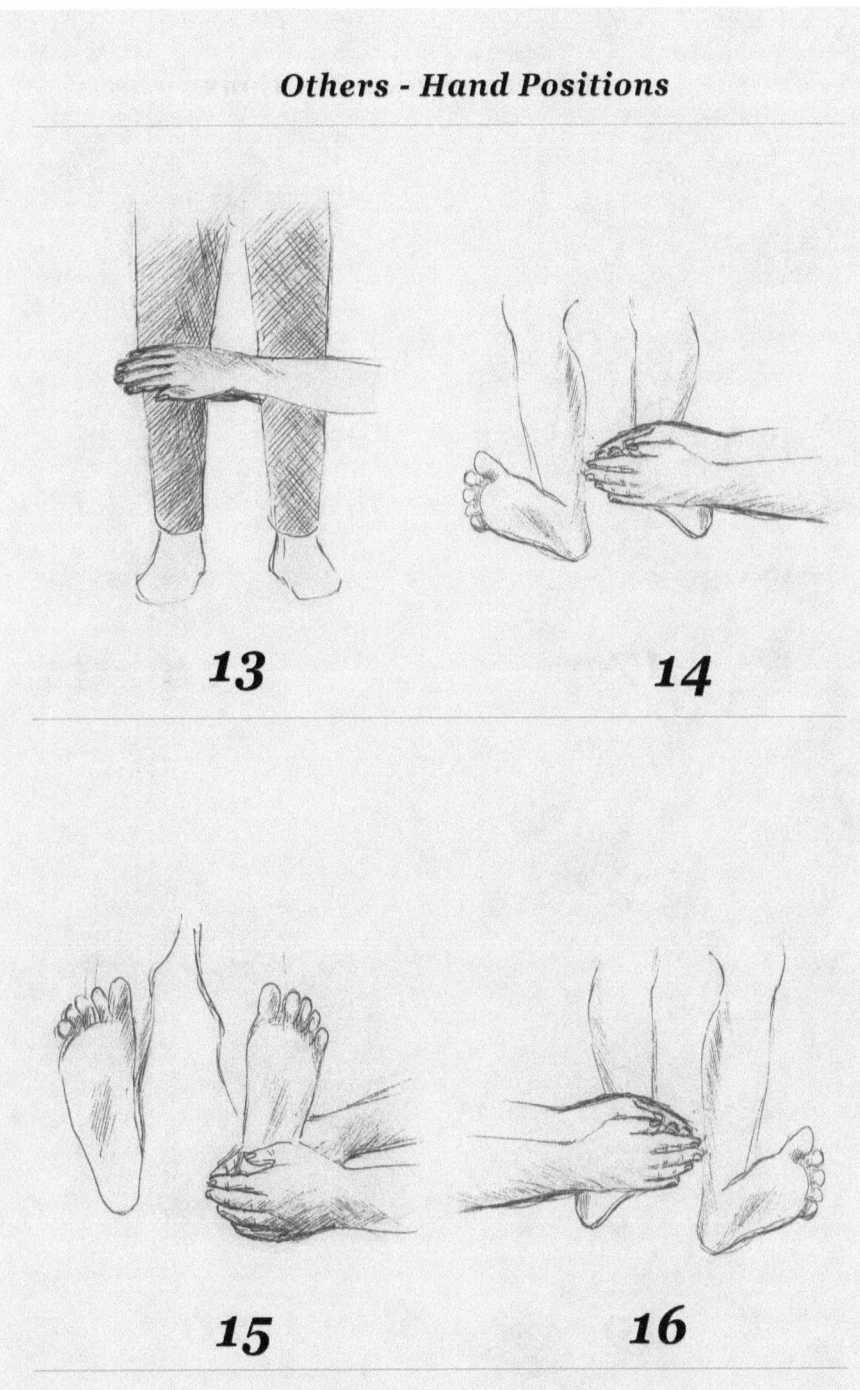

13

14

15

16

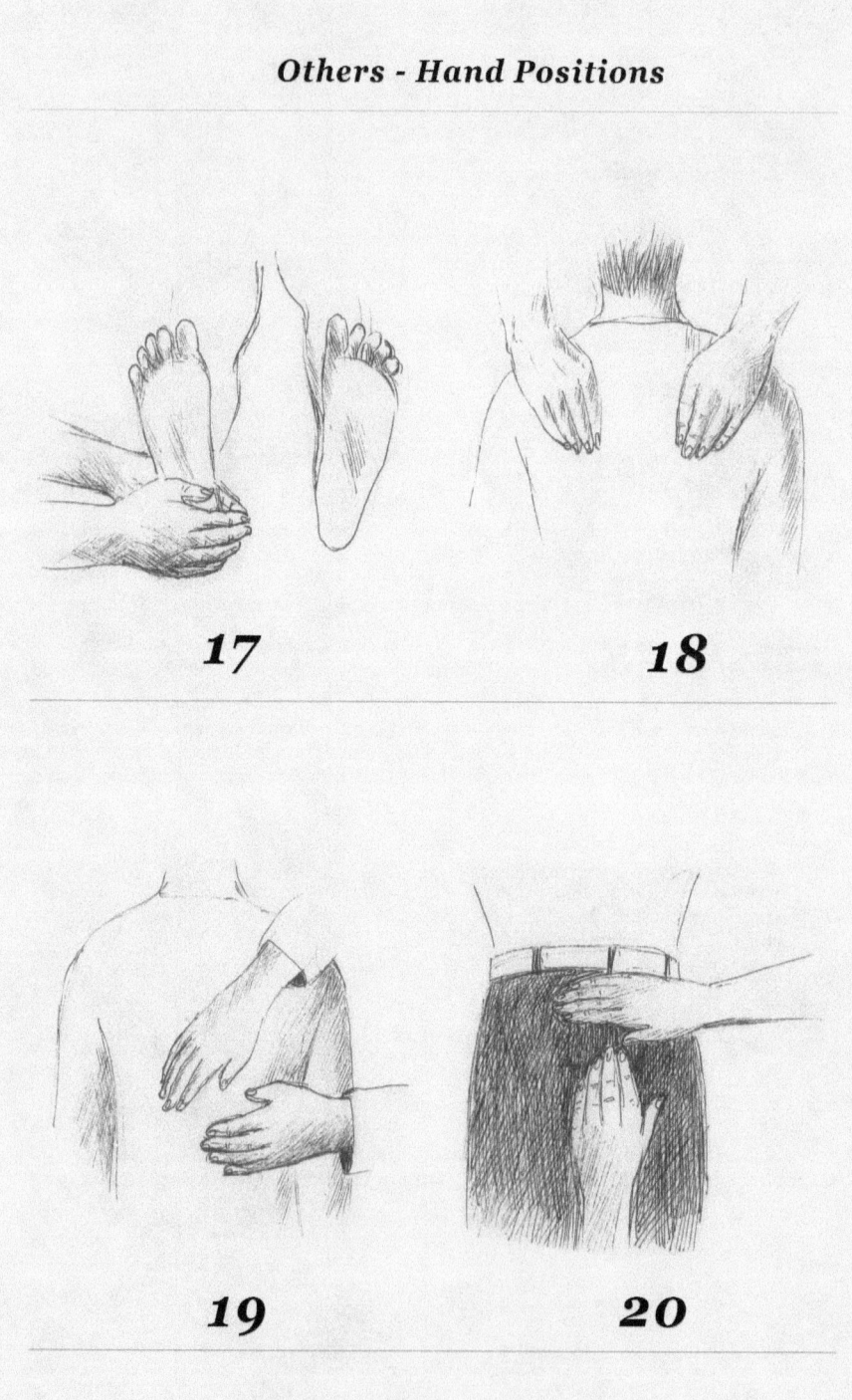

Others - Hand Positions

17

18

19

20

Reiki Manuals

Level Two & Three

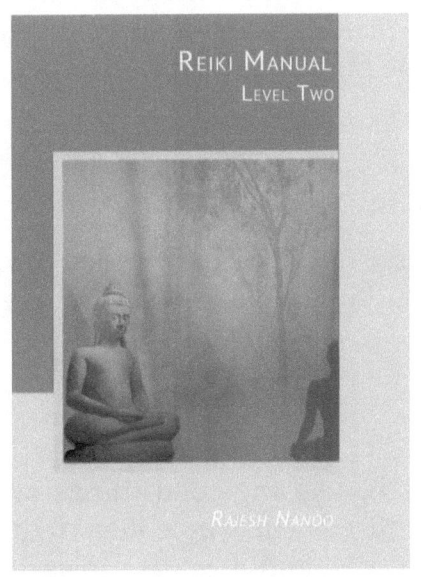
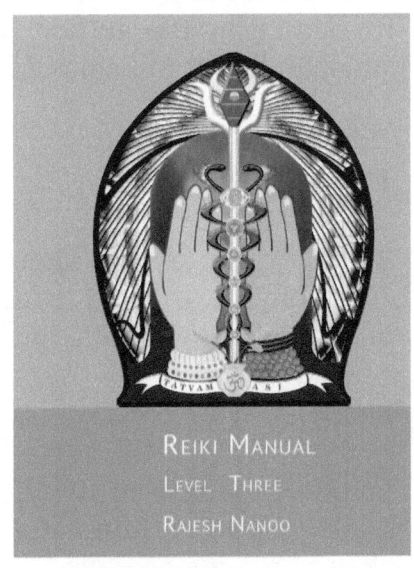

Paperbacks and EBooks are available in Createspace, Amazon, Lulu, Smashwords etc. Contact author website for more details.

www.rajeshnanoo.com

Other Books

1. The Cave Of Wisdom

The Book contains the gist of mystical teachings from Upanishads, Zen, Sufism, Kabbala, Buddhism and Taoism. Along with this, it covers the very essence of Semitic philosophy that is spread through Christianity, Islam and Judaism.

The book has many verses and stories of Upanishad exclusively translated by the author. The principal ideologies said by Upanishad Saints are shared in the book.

2. Wine Of Words

This book contains 100 short verses of progressive ideology. These thoughts aroused from Zen, Sufi, and Kabbalistic wisdom baptized in Vedantic doctrines.

3. Be......

31 mindful matters to middle path. All the good things are possible only when mind feels inspired. The whole idea of the book is to make people to be reflective and receptive towards every situations of life.

4. Reiki Sutras

Reiki the vibrational energy medicine when emitted through hands of Healer whose mind meditating on subtle love realms have the potential to relax, rejuvenate and renovate any human body and subtle bodies. The book explores the pillars and healing methodology of Reiki, which was built from the foundation laid by Saints in Indian Tantra and Lamas from Buddhism.